THE
REFLEXOLOGY
HANDBOOK

THE REFLEXOLOGY HANDBOOK

A COMPLETE GUIDE

Laura Norman
with Thomas Cowan

PIATKUS

Authors' and Publisher's Note

This book is not intended to replace the advice of a trained health professional. If you know, or suspect, that you have a health problem, you should consult a health professional.

Copyright © 1988 by Laura Norman
Illustrations copyright © by Laura Norman and Ivey Barry
Chapter illustrations by Paul Gorham
Designed by Bonni Leon

This edition first published in
Great Britain in 1989 by
Judy Piatkus (Publishers) Ltd of
5 Windmill Street, London W1

Reprinted 1990 (twice)

British Library Cataloguing in Publication Data

Norman, Laura
    The reflexology handbook.
    1. Man. Therapy. Use of reflex massage of feet
    I. Title   II. Cowan, Thomas
    615.8'22

    ISBN 0-86188-886-3
    ISBN 0-86188-912-6 (pbk)

Printed and bound in Great Britain by
The Bath Press, Bath, Avon

This book is lovingly dedicated to my husband, Warren Berland, whose confidence in me and my work has been a constant source of inspiration. His steadfast love and encouragement made it possible for me to write this book.

For all of your love, support, encouragement, ideas, word processing, editing, proofreading, and artwork.

Ivey Barry
Adella Basayne-Smith
Deborah Bergman
William Bergman
Warren Berland
Lonny Black
Dwight Byers
Victor Caamano
Dale Cabrera
George Chirayus
Connie Clausen
Tom Cowan
Toni Lee Curry
Enoch Davis
Joe DeLeo
Jessie Green

Barbara Gess
Elaine Hyams Koelmel
Richard Johnson
Jane Kerns
Bonni Leon
My mom, Irene Mazur Mahler
Eugene Mahler
Holly Papa
Jan Shapiro
Joseph Siegel
Lorraine Simone
Hugh Slater
Terri Soller
Natalie Stanley
Ann Williams

CONTENTS

Foreword   9

Introduction   12

ONE   Why Reflexology   15

TWO   Learning Reflexology   47

THREE   Doing Reflexology   97

FOUR   The Nature of Stress   127

FIVE   Getting Ahead: Reflexology at Work and School   133

SIX   Sole Mates: Couples' Reflexology   151

SEVEN   The Cycles of Life: Reflexology for Women   169

EIGHT   Growing Feet: Children's Reflexology   193

NINE   After Walking Many Miles: Reflexology in the Golden Years   219

TEN   The Active Life: Reflexology and Athletics   241

ELEVEN   Getting Unhooked: Overcoming Addictions with Reflexology   255

TWELVE   The Final Steps: Reflexology and Terminal Illness   267

THIRTEEN   Using Reflexology to Strengthen the Body's Systems   269

FOURTEEN   Reflexology and the Health Care Professions   283

FIFTEEN   Table of Common Conditions   285

Index   331

FOREWORD

Marvelous, simply marvelous, is the way I feel about Laura Norman and reflexology. Actually, there is no difference between Laura Norman and reflexology, since she is so dedicated to her work and to the expansion of this wonderful healing art.

I have been fortunate to work with Laura, and it is always exciting to see her functioning at 100 percent, committed to bringing better health to people through reflexology. I, too, am a health practitioner, and am aware of the value that a personality has in the healing process. Laura's pleasant, honest personality, coupled with her magical hands and commitment, make her a leader and true pioneer in the healing field of reflexology. You can be assured that if Laura works on you, you will leave feeling ecstatic and with two "happy soles."

Because reflexology brings total relaxation, it can complement any health care work. Considering its therapeutic effects, there are few contraindications to its application. Therefore, one of Laura's goals is to reach as many soles as possible, hoping to bring fulfillment and excellence back into their lives by providing a stress reliever.

From a purely anatomical viewpoint, each foot has thirty-three joints and is innervated by thousands of nerves. By using specific reflexology techniques, one directly affects the nervous system in a very positive, relaxing way. When the body is relaxed and the nervous system stimulated, healing has a perfect opportunity to take place. For, as I have seen, healing comes from the inside out.

I have only the highest regard for Laura and the work of reflexology. I personally have received benefits from this science and recommend it to my patients. So, if you are now being introduced to reflexology, or are an advanced student, know that you have embarked on the study of an ancient healing art that will definitely continue to grow. Good luck on your course of study and in its application.

Anthony Buonocore, D.C.

As a physician and health educator concerned with preventive medicine, methods to naturally enhance the immune system, and other self-healing mechanisms, I have become convinced of the value of reflexology because of my patients' reports of their beneficial responses to this gentle healing art. The benefits of reflexology are enhanced by Laura Norman's commitment, devotion, and love for people. In my opinion, these above all other qualities set the standard of personal and professional excellence that will characterize the true healing and medical professions of the New Age.

William L. Bergman, M.D.

In the foot, we find a fascinating focus for the understanding and promulgation of human health. The condition of the foot is a reflection of the status of the major body systems: skin, musculoskeletal, secretory, nervous, and circulatory. The art and science of reflexology further augments the role of the foot in providing a means to improve the human condition.

The methods I have learned at the Laura Norman Reflexology Center have been invaluable in my clinical practice of podiatric medicine, surgery, and biomechanics. The methods described herein can improve nervous and circulatory function and can help the body achieve a higher degree of homeostasis. Intrinsic benefits for the foot include the ability to accelerate the dissolution of postoperative and posttraumatic scar tissue and adhesions. In addition, reflexology techniques may mobilize, and thereby assist in, the elimination of certain crystalline waste products that accumulate in the foot.

Certainly, one of the most profoundly valuable benefits of Ms. Norman's techniques is the ability to help the patient achieve a state of deep relaxation. Through this process of deep relaxation, a better posture and gait may be achieved. Thus we see improvement in total body function.

It is my hope that my colleagues in allopathic medicine will begin to join the quest for health by accepting Ms. Norman's techniques and applying them in a broad range of human disorders.

My congratulations to Ms. Laura Norman upon the publication of this landmark text.

Clifford B. Levy, D.P.M.

Many different means of pain control and stress relief have been tried throughout the centuries. In spite of gigantic technical progress, including flights to the moon and computerized biomechanics, progress in certain areas of medical science has not kept up with the industrial revolution.

Moreover, we are discovering that certain methods which were applied hundreds of years ago are coming back to life and being used more and more. We are now openly and proudly learning from ancient naturopathic and oriental methods. Next to acupuncture, acupressure, and different types of body therapies, reflexology is one of the most convincing and applicable methods of controlling different types of pain and stress.

Reflexology is using authentic anatomical knowledge in combination with skillful hand work, applying deep and light pressure over the complex nerve-ending network of human feet.

As a medical doctor specializing in neurology, and from both my medical knowledge and my personal experience, I can only give my full approval to this old-new method. I hope that more physicians will accept reflexology as part of their standard treatment modality.

My congratulations to Laura Norman, a pioneer in reflexology, who with her warm devotion, charm, and knowledge, can teach us to practice truly holistic medicine.

Vera Zablozki, M.D.

INTRODUCTION

In 1983 I spoke about reflexology at the Whole Life Expo in New York City to a small audience of eighteen people, ten of whom were my family and friends. Just three years later I again spoke at the New York Expo to a standing-room-only audience in a hall that held hundreds. The dramatic rise in interest in reflexology is a sign of our times. We are becoming more health conscious in ways that were never dreamed of a generation or two ago. We are discovering that health is truly holistic, that we are well only if our bodies *and* minds cooperate in creating a state of well-being for the entire person.

Mind, body, and emotions are intimately interwoven, so much so that what we do for any part of ourselves impacts on the rest of our being. For we are not made up of parts. We are wholes. What I have found, as have thousands of others in recent years, is that reflexology is one of the best methods for bringing health and harmony to the total person.

When I first began my career as a reflexologist in the early 1970s, the climate was even more challenging. Very few people had heard of reflexology, even though it has been around since the early years of the century. As my practice grew and I began talking about reflexology on radio and television shows, and in the leading magazines that deal with health and personal improvement issues, word eventually spread. People were eager, even hungry, for the good news: that relaxation, peace of mind, energy, and a body that functions harmoniously and efficiently, as it was meant to do, can be part of everyone's life.

And how is this possible? Through reflexology, a specific type of steady, even pressure to the feet that produces dynamic healing and relaxation in all parts of the body. Results have been truly startling in overcoming or easing a broad range of problems, from chronic ailments and weight and stress disorders to women's labor pains.

I have been privileged to be the bearer of these good tidings, to announce to hundreds of thousands of people that not only is it fun and rewarding to receive the benefits of reflexology, but it is even more rewarding to be the reflexologist who can bring these gifts to others.

I first learned about reflexology when I was a student at Boston University in the early 1970s. Like many in my generation, I experimented with the various mind/body disciplines that were slowly coming into the mainstream of American life: shiatsu, massage, yoga, transcendental meditation, visualization techniques, and the many different types of diets and exercise therapies. While each has something beneficial to offer, none seemed to have such a positive, encompassing effect on me as reflexology. In reflexology I found a method to improve communication, trust, peace, and love, and to instill deep relaxation and an incredible sense of well-being—or as most of my clients put it, "feeling great all over." Truly, reflexology touched me deeply on physical, emotional, mental, and profound spiritual levels that I did not experience with any other holistic discipline.

I studied privately with several reflexologists in the Boston area and eventually decided to become a certified reflexologist. I then contacted Dwight Byers, who has done more than anyone to promote the reflexology method developed by his aunt, Eunice Ingham. Without his untiring, pioneering work to educate both the American and the international publics, as well as the traditional medical professions, about reflexology as an alternative health care discipline, the field of reflexology would not have achieved the giant strides toward recognition and acceptance that it has in recent years.

After completing the professional training course in the Original Ingham Method, I began practicing in New York City. Early in my career, while working in an institution with emotionally disturbed and multiply handicapped children, many of whom were labeled as "hopeless," I watched reflexology help these special children become calmer, happier, more alert, and able to learn faster. The practical value became even more apparent to me as I worked with other children, business executives, athletes, creative and performing artists, senior citizens, and fellow health practitioners. Because I have seen how reflexology can revolutionize the lives of so many different types of people, I wanted to write a book on the specific, practical ways that reflexology can become part of one's life.

Over the years my own work has evolved into the most extensive, in-depth program for training professional reflexologists. I have been associated with physicians, surgeons, podiatrists, chiropractors, gynecologists, dentists, optometrists, and psychotherapists, and am continually encouraged by the praise of these experts for the many benefits of reflexology and by their recommendations to their own patients and clients to discover it for themselves. My former students are currently practicing all across the nation. Today thousands of people put their feet first by making reflexology an important part of their lives, receiving reflexology and giving it to others, enriching their relationships with family, friends, and loved ones.

What I love most about my work is to see people experience results—a sense of wholeness, well-being, and revitalized energy. People afflicted with illnesses and health problems begin to heal. Others begin to experience their inner life forces more intensely, freeing the creative spirit from inner blockages, setting them on a path of self-expression.

I consider myself privileged to have watched a dream come true over the last eighteen years. What I experienced back in my college days—the total relaxation and serenity that allows one to live life more creatively, energetically, and at peace with oneself—is now being experienced by countless men, women, and children across the country. Today reflexology is better known and accepted by lay people as well as by the medical professions. But there is still a long way to go before it enjoys full recognition and its rightful place among the healing arts and the health care delivery system.

Yes, I have watched a dream come true, and the dream continues. I would like to see reflexology become a household word and to establish reflexology centers in all the major cities of the country in order to make reflexology more accessible to people everywhere. *The Reflexology Handbook* is the first step in doing just that.

You will find that this book is unlike any other book on reflexology. It is about people, the stages of life and the activities that are important to the quality of life: work, play, parenting, nurturing. Here you will learn techniques—tools, if you will—for being with people and relating to them in warm and inspiring ways. Giving reflexology deepens relationships, inspires trust, and brings people together, making communication easier and more open.

I hope that as you read this book you will be inspired to learn reflexology and begin practicing it on yourself and with others. There are many ways to incorporate reflexology into your daily living. As you will discover, there is a place for reflexology in everyone's life, young or old, male or female, single or married, healthy or not. Reflexology is not like aspirin or cough syrup, a remedy to be pulled out of the medicine cabinet only when you are feeling ill. No, reflexology is also for the strong and vigorous, the busy, energetic professional man or woman whose life is constantly on the go. Perhaps it is even more important for healthy people to make it part of their lives—for everyone needs balance, relaxation, moments of reflection and serenity to get in touch with their deepest selves and experience the peace and well-being that lies within.

CHAPTER ONE

WHY REFLEXOLOGY

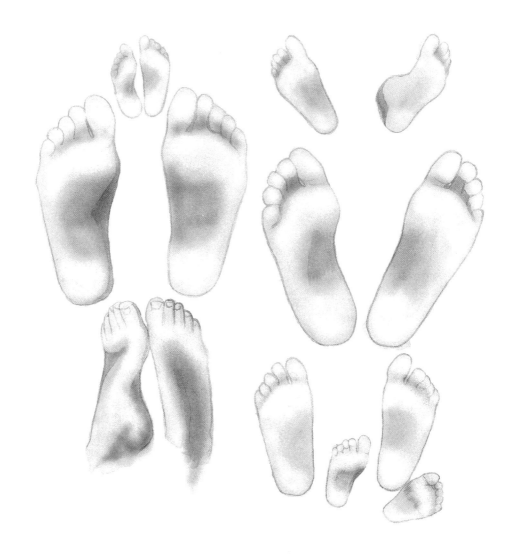

Touching is an intimate act. Whether it is a hearty handshake or a tender embrace, when we touch another person, something happens between us. A relationship begins. If we continue to reach out to each other, the relationship grows. We share and exchange, and we are enriched. We may give presents, meals, time, interest, or love, but we are really always giving the same gift—ourselves. Reflexology offers the perfect opportunity for giving the gift of ourselves in a way that brings health and well-being to those we care about. My husband Warren and I know immediately when the other is having a stressful day, and we also know exactly what to do about it. Grab a foot! Within minutes we can dispel each other's stress or anxiety.

Touching the feet. We hardly ever do it. Some people even manage to put on their shoes and socks without really coming into contact with their feet. This is one of the reasons reflexology can revolutionize our lives. It is something we don't ordinarily do! It is special, something out of the ordinary. It provides a valuable opportunity for us to let go of the usual problems and activities of the day and relax with someone we enjoy being with and then just "be." Most of us live lives that have very little time for this. We live in a sea of noise, deadlines, interruptions, worries, responsibilities, and distractions that keep us from being with those we love. Reflexology can provide a quiet island in the course of each day where we can get together, stop the commotion, take stock of what is really important, and renew ourselves so we can return to our busy worlds with more energy and enthusiasm.

Reflexology can be the first step in discovering other ways to live happier and healthier lives. By putting your feet first with reflexology, you'll realize how good you can feel; and you'll want to learn how to find other quiet islands for taking care of yourself and your loved ones. Studies have shown that people who incorporate activities like meditation, reading, absorbing hobbies, or physical exercise into their schedules—either alone or with someone else—tend to be healthier, happier, and more efficient in all areas of their lives. Reflexology can be your introduction to these kinds of relaxing and renewing moments. So take the first step by putting your feet first. Let your feet not only *take* steps but *become* the first step in leading you to discover other ways to live more fully.

WHAT EXACTLY IS REFLEXOLOGY?

Reflexology is a method for activating the healing powers of the body. It is both old and new. From ancient texts, illustrations, and artifacts, we know that the early Chinese, Japanese, Indians, Russians, and Egyptians worked on the feet to promote good health. Today many of these same techniques have been developed into a modern scientific method called reflexology. What joins the ancients with the moderns is the long-established principle that there are energy zones that run throughout the body and reflex areas in the feet that correspond to all the major organs, glands, and body parts.

In the early years of the twentieth century, Dr. William Fitzgerald developed the modern zone theory of the human body, arguing that parts of the body correspond to other parts and offering as proof the fact that applying pressure to one area anesthetized a corresponding area. Dr. Edwin Bowers, Fitzgerald's colleague, used a dramatic demonstration to convince others of the theory's validity. He showed that he could stick a pin into a volunteer's face without causing pain if he first applied pressure to the point in the person's hand which corresponded to that area of the face.

In the 1930s, Eunice Ingham, a physiotherapist for Dr. Joseph Shelby Riley, who was also a student and advocate of the theory, used zone therapy in her work with patients. She concluded that since the zones ran throughout the body and could be accessed anywhere, some areas might be more accessible and effective than others. She was right. The feet were the most responsive areas for working the zones because they were extremely sensitive. Eventually, she mapped the entire body onto the feet and discovered that an alternating pressure on the various points had therapeutic effects far beyond the limited use to which zone therapy had been previously employed, namely, reduction of pain. And so reflexology was born.

Modern reflexology is both a science and an art. As a science, it requires careful study, faithful practice, a sound knowledge of the techniques, and skill. And yet as one of the healing arts, reflexology yields the best results when the reflexologist works with dedication, patience, focused intention, and above all, loving care.

Before we look at how and why reflexology works, let's consider its many benefits.

Reflexology reduces stress and induces deep relaxation.

Stress cannot be avoided. We live *with* it and *in* it everyday. In itself, stress is neither good nor bad. Playing tennis or giving a dinner party is stressful and yet exhilarating and fun. Stress becomes a problem, however, when we fail to manage it well, especially the stress that results from problems, frustrations, overwork, and worry. When we don't handle stress well, the body's defenses break down and we become more susceptible to illness and disease. It's been estimated that over seventy-five percent of all illness is stress-related. Reflexology reduces stress by generating deep, tranquil relaxation. Many of my clients routinely fall asleep during a reflexology session and testify on waking that the thirty or forty minutes of sleep were more beneficial and restorative than a full night of restless sleep. We all know how good it feels to lie down in the middle of a busy day. But lying down is just the first step. Beyond that lie the deep realms of relaxation and peace that help the body balance itself and allow healing energy to flow smoothly and gently throughout.

Every part of the body is operated by messages carried back and forth along neural pathways. Stimulation of sensory nerve endings sends information to the spinal cord and brain. The brain and spinal cord send instructions to the organs and muscles. The neural pathways are both living tissue and electrical channels, and can be impinged upon or polluted by many factors. When neural pathways are impaired, nerve function is impeded—messages are delivered slowly and unreliably, or not at all, and body processes operate at less than optimum levels. The reflexologist stimulates more than 7,000 nerves when touching the feet, and encourages the opening and clearing of neural pathways.

Reflexology improves circulation.

We all know how important it is for blood to flow freely throughout the body, carrying oxygen and nutrients to all the cells that make up the tissues of the body and removing waste products of metabolism, and other toxins. What many of us aren't aware of is that the blood vessels contract and relax in this process and that their resiliency is most important for proper functioning. Stress and tension tighten up the cardiovascular system and restrict blood flow. Circulation becomes sluggish. By reducing stress and tension, reflexology allows the miles of cardiovascular vessels to conduct the flow of blood naturally and easily.

Reflexology cleanses the body of toxins and impurities.

The body has built-in mechanisms for cleansing itself, mainly the lymphatic, excretory, and integumentary systems (i.e., the lymph nodes, the kidneys and colon, and the skin). If these become blocked or function improperly, toxins and waste matter build up. A healthy body is like a healthy home: You have to take the garbage out regularly. By deepening relaxation, reflexology causes all the systems of the body to function more efficiently, including those that eliminate waste products.

Reflexology balances the whole system.

The technical term is *homeostasis* and it means being in a dynamic state of balance. To me it means togetherness and centeredness. The thousands of parts and areas of the body, each functioning according to its own laws and purposes, together make up only one body. For the body to be healthy, everything must work together. If one part is out of whack, other parts suffer. To keep the body running harmoniously, a tune-up is often needed. As after a motor tune-up, the end result is a machine that runs smoothly, with all its parts contributing synergistically.

Reflexology revitalizes energy.

Energy is very personal. We all experience it in our own ways. You know when your "juices are flowing" and when they're not. Sometimes energy is exciting and invigorating; at other times it is calm and restful. We each experience our energy levels in personal and subtle ways. But one thing is certain: Energy flows. It circulates consciously and unconsciously throughout the body on a physical, emotional, and mental level. There is also an energy of the spirit that is just as crucial to overall well-being as physical or mental energy. Like the old metaphysical issue of the One and the Many, there may be only one source of Energy in the universe, and each type we experience is an expression of it. Be that as it may, energy needs to be revitalized periodically. According to polarity theory, it must also flow unimpeded between the negative and positive poles that every atom and cell contains. Or in Oriental thought, the yin and yang energy currents must complement each other. In whatever terms make sense to you, feeling good and alive requires sufficient energy. By relaxing and opening up energy pathways, reflexology revitalizes the body and supplies it with energy on all levels.

When my grandmother was suffering from cancer in her eighties, she was usually weak and had very little energy to perform the normal daily activities of a woman her age. I gave her regular reflexology sessions and she always responded with renewed strength and energy. Doctors who treated her were amazed at what she could do when reflexology was an ongoing part of her health care. Although the cancer did not go into remission, her energy levels and natural vitality improved considerably.

Reflexology is preventive health care.

Preventive health care is becoming more important as we realize the health-threatening dangers of our environment: stress, fatigue, chemical additives in food, polluted water supplies, radioactivity, and poor air quality, to name only a few. The added strain on everyone's immune system today should warn us to find time to unwind and relax, because the immune system functions at its peak only when a person successfully manages the stressful situations of daily life. The immune system also responds synergistically, relying on other bodily processes to maintain its own lines of defense. Only when the body is well balanced is a person in good shape to ward off illness.

My clients who are teachers and parents tell me that they are less suscepti-ble to catching colds during the flu seasons even though their kids sneeze and cough around them all the time. Adults don't have immunity to the bugs that children carry around. But reflexology seems to help in bolstering im-munological defenses, and so they catch fewer colds. Children get fewer colds too when they receive reflexology.

Reflexology stimulates creativity and productivity.

Very few of us can perform at our best if we are sluggish and tired. Like exercise, reflexology restores mental alertness and improves the attention span. By reducing tensions and calming the mind, we are free to think our best thoughts, come up with our best ideas, and work longer and with greater clarity at difficult tasks. Each session provides the quiet time so necessary to let new ideas gestate. As a pick-me-up in the middle of the day or in the late afternoon, reflexology can send you back to work or into the evening with the mental energy you need to be creative and productive.

Reflexology nurtures relationships.

Reflexology can unite two people in a special, intimate relationship and strengthen that relationship every time you do it. Eventually the wonderful chemistry between the two of you spreads to others. When you feel good, others respond. My clients go back to their offices more patient and tolerant of co-workers, and pretty soon their presence changes the whole work environment. Feeling good is contagious!

Reflexology rewards the practitioner.

All body workers and healers will tell you that their work is rewarding, not just because they help others to feel good and enjoy better health but because when they act as a channel for healing energy, the circuit completes itself by bringing health and well-being to them too. They feel grounded and centered; their attention is focused and concentrated even as the recipient relaxes and becomes centered. In fact, just looking forward to giving a reflexology session has a calming effect on me. I know that for the next hour I'll be centered and grounded and can forget about the rest of the world for a while. Afterward, the reflexologist feels a great sense of satisfaction, and receives "strokes" of another kind in the gratitude and thank-yous lavished by the client.

HOW DOES REFLEXOLOGY WORK?

Since ancient times, healers have employed various methodologies to strengthen and balance the energy flow. Many of these systems, including acupuncture, shiatsu, and reflexology, agree that this energy flows in zones or meridians throughout the body. Reflexologists specify that there are ten energy zones that run the length of the body from head to toe—five on each side of the body ending in each foot and running down the arms into the tips of the fingers. Not only do these zones run lengthwise, but they pass *through the body,* so that a zone located on the front of the body can also be reached from behind. All the organs and parts of the body lie along one or more of these zones.

The ten energy zones of the body.

Each zone can be considered a channel for the intangible life energy, called *chi* or *qi* in oriental medicine and martial arts. Stimulating or "working" any zone in the foot by applying pressure with the thumbs and fingers affects the entire zone throughout the body. For example, working a zone on the foot along which the kidneys lie will release vital energy that may be blocked somewhere else in that zone, such as in the eyes. Working the kidney reflex area on the foot will therefore revitalize and balance the entire zone and improve functioning of the organ.

The actual physical mechanism that controls the ten zones in the body and feet is not fully understood. That it works is proven every day, but exactly how it works is still a mystery. There are sound, reputable theories, however, suggesting that good health depends on balance, equilibrium, the natural functioning of all the body systems—that we call homeostasis. Excessive stress disrupts this balance. In fact, the stress reaction is a very primitive response to a situation perceived as dangerous or threatening. It has been called the "fight or flight response" because our spontaneous reaction is to gear up the body and emotions either to fight off the attacker or run for our lives. The problem for contemporary people living in our modern civilization is that it isn't considered civilized to fight and there's no place to run! Unfortunately our adrenal glands don't know this, so the heartbeat becomes more rapid, the digestive system shuts down, and a chain of other physical reactions occur to prepare us for the looming "catastrophe." But often we do nothing except bottle it up and repress it. Eventually, the stress buildup "explodes" internally by knocking some part of our system out of balance.

Reflexology alleviates the effects of stress by inducing deep relaxation, placing us in a "safe space," and allowing the nervous system to calm down and function more normally. Circulation proceeds smoothly, blood flow is improved, and oxygen reaches all the cells. We are no longer activated for fight or flight. The body seeks homeostasis, and healing can take place. The person experiences a sense of well-being at all levels.

As in acupuncture or shiatsu, energy pathways are opened up, and the subtle energy that accompanies neurological and circulatory functioning can do its work. Order and harmony are restored. The body is normalized as the seven energy centers, known in Eastern medicine as the *chakras,* are unblocked. The body returns to its natural rhythms. Energy flows. The body, mind, and spirit are brought back into balance.

WHY THE FEET?

We live in a holographic universe. The energy, information, knowledge, and wisdom of the All is contained in every cell and particle. Every day physicists are discovering just how interrelated the cosmos really is, and yet these discoveries would be considered old hat to the mystics and seers of the past and present. Evidence of this interweaving of All Life is all around us. We don't need rocks from the moon, shells from the ocean depths, or DNA material from the living body to see the correspondences. Just look at your feet.

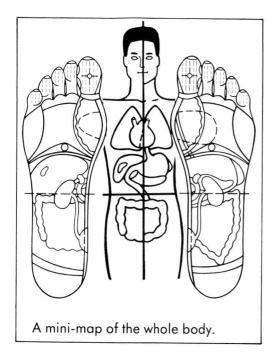

A mini-map of the whole body.

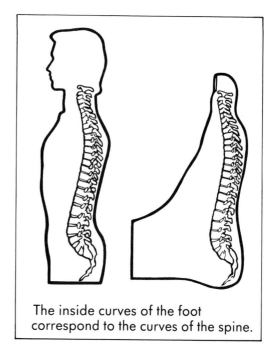

The inside curves of the foot correspond to the curves of the spine.

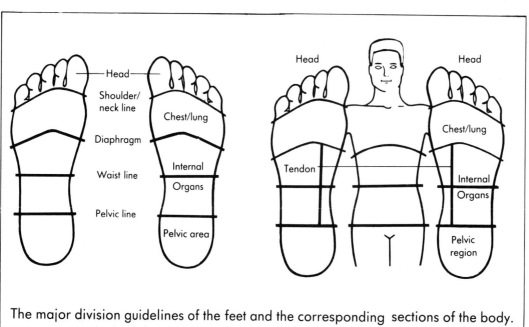

The major division guidelines of the feet and the corresponding sections of the body.

As you can see in the illustration, the feet are a perfect microcosm or mini-map of the whole body. All the organs, glands and body parts represented in the foot are laid out in the same arrangement as in the body. Even the inside curve of the foot corresponds to the natural curves in the spine. The toes are like little heads. The ridge beneath them on the top part of the ball of the foot is a natural shoulder or neck line. The waist line tightens inward as it should! In fact, you can tell whether someone is high- or low-waisted just by checking out the waist line on the foot.

Other parts of the body exhibit these same correspondences, but less obviously. The hand, the ear, even the iris of the eye contain reflex points for the entire body. But these points are more specific in the feet; and because they are more spread out and accessible, they are easier to work with. We would need microscopic equipment to stimulate distinct reflex points in a cell. On the feet we can use our hands.

In fact, the feet are remarkably sensitive even though most of us would probably think that our hands beat out the feet when it comes to sensitivity. But not so. We are more familiar with our hands and know how to use them for sensing and manipulating the world. We love our hands, but we don't always love our feet. Nevertheless, the feet are actually more sensitive and receptive, partly because of the wealth of nerve endings and partly because we keep them covered and protected. I'm sure you've had the experience of drawing bathwater, testing it carefully with your hand before getting in, only to find that when your foot—or big toe—touches the water, it suddenly got too hot! No, it was always too hot—for your foot if not for your hand.

The feet are also distant enough from the torso that most people are not threatened by having someone work on them. The head, heart, lung and trunk areas of the human body seem more private than the limbs or extremities. Since many people are not used to having someone else lay hands on their bodies, they can be self-conscious about having these parts touched. It helps them relax if the area being worked on is not too close to the "vital center."

The foot is also ideally shaped and sized for the human hand. We can hold a foot naturally and easily. It's neither too big nor too small. When receiving a reflexology treatment a person has a reassuring sense that the reflexologist is in control, as the hands can support the foot and touch it all over most of the time. It's not like massage, where the practitioner works on one part of the body, leaves it to move on to another, and may or may not return to the first area. In reflexology the receiver has a sense that even though the reflexologist's hands move around on the feet, it is the entire foot that is being worked on continuously. This is very reassuring and the effect is more holistic.

The feet ground us, literally and figuratively. They are our contact with the earth and the energies that flow through it. They are our base, our foundation. A steady foot means stability and security. When we "lose our footing," we loose our equilibrium and sense of balance. Our body—and mind—know all this whether we think about it consciously or not. On a deeper spiritual level, we also know that this grounding contact with the earth is rooted in who we are as people, a spirit incarnate in living flesh, that we are made up of the elements just as the world around us is. English-speaking people live with an important insight whether we consciously hear it or not: We walk on our soles/souls.

There are some important biological and anatomical reasons for working with the feet. They are farthest from the heart, where circulation tends to stagnate. People with chronically poor circulation often have tender or swollen hands and feet. It is good to stimulate and encourage blood flow to these extremities. What's more, gravity pulls toxins downward. Inorganic waste materials such as uric acid and calcium crystals can build up in the bottoms of the feet. An experienced reflexologist can actually feel these deposits with his or her hands and break up these crystals with reflexology techniques. In general, circulation can stagnate in the feet. Kneading the feet during reflexology breaks up the deposits and improves circulation in the feet themselves.

Last, we owe it to our feet to do something good for them. Of all the parts of the body, they take a real beating. They bear our weight, they are under considerable tension, and we cram them into shoe styles (and sizes) that are not always best for them. Between concrete, inappropriate shoes, and poor postural habits, the muscles and joints of the modern foot receive little sustenance. In fact, many people experience tremendous daily pain in their feet, and tune it out of their conscious awareness with a neurological process known as *adaptation*. Yet even without awareness, constant pain takes its toll in muscle tension elsewhere in the body—especially in the neck and shoulders—and in increased fatigue and irritability. Clients often express amazement at how much their feet need reflexology and how little they realized it.

We abuse our feet. You know how good it feels to take off your shoes and socks and wiggle your toes, let the air get to them, even put them up. It feels wonderful to free your feet. Reflexology is foot freedom and more.

WHAT REFLEXOLOGY IS NOT

There is a lot of misinformation about reflexology, as there is about many of the non-Western methods of healing. In general, reflexology is not massage and it is not medicine as practiced by Western-trained physicians. In plain language, it is not a foot massage and it is not a medical treatment. First and foremost, reflexologists do not diagnose illness, nor do they practice medicine. Only licensed physicians are allowed to do that according to law. Neither does a reflexologist treat specific diseases. Even though most of my clients tell me very specifically what their problems are—and when you work on family members and friends you may know what ailments they suffer from—we never proceed as if a reflexology session is going to cure these problems. We spend extra time working the reflex area on the foot that corresponds to the body part that is troubled, but our work cannot be classified as medical treatment as such.

From what we have already discussed, it should be plain that reflexology works with subtle energy flows, revitalizing the body so that the natural internal healing mechanisms of the body can do their own work. As a matter of fact, people do attest to better health, even sometimes a marked reduction or even disappearance of the ailment. But it was not the reflexologist nor the session that cured. Only the body cures.

The reflexologist is a channel of healing. The laying on of hands and the specific techniques for applying pressure to the feet create the channels for healing energy to circulate to all parts of the body. No instruments or gadgets are ever used, only the hands. When practiced in conjunction with sound medical advice from your physician, reflexology facilitates healing.

FEET: THE MIRROR OF THE BODY

Each foot represents half of the body, the left and right foot corresponding to the left and right side of the body. (See illustration.)

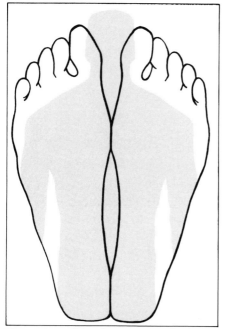

The soles of the feet mirror the body.

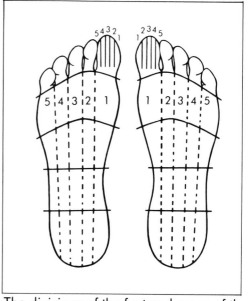

The divisions of the feet and areas of the body to which they refer.

Here is a list of the divisions of the feet and the areas of the body to which they correspond:

TOES	=	Head and neck
BALLS OF FEET (METATARSALS)	=	Chest, lung area, shoulder
ARCH (UPPER PART)	=	Diaphragm to waist area
ARCH (LOWER PART)	=	Waist to pelvic area
HEEL	=	Pelvic area/sciatic nerve
INNER FOOT (MEDIAL SIDE)	=	Spine
OUTER FOOT (LATERAL SIDE)	=	Arm, shoulder, hip, leg, knee, lower back
ANKLE AREA	=	Pelvic area, reproductive organs

Using these divisions and the five zones, you can locate any area of the body on the mini-map of the foot. Let's say someone indicates a pain by pointing to the area just beneath the rib cage on the right and a little above the waist. Without knowing exactly what the problem is, you can locate the specific area on the foot. Since the pain is on the right, the reflex point would be on the right foot between the diaphragm line and the waist line and along zone 5. A reflex point is a specific area or point on the foot that corresponds to another part of the body. When stimulated by the thumbs or fingers, there is a response to the stimulus in another part of the body.

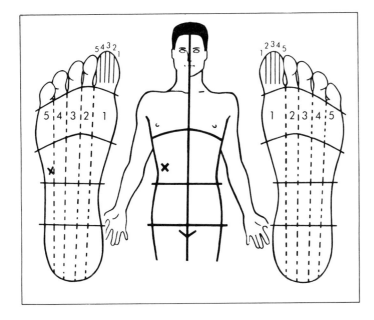

Use the divisions and zones on the foot to locate a reflex area in the body.

You will also notice another guideline for locating specific points on the foot. This is the long tendon that runs vertically down the arch between zones 1 and 2. To find the tendon, pull the toes back to stretch the skin tighter across the arch. The tendon will come forward. It is important not to apply pressure on the tendon itself when you are working this area, because doing so is painful. Always hop over the tendon when you are thumb walking in this area (described in the following chapter). As you become better acquainted with the foot, you'll begin to think of certain points as being either to the left or right of this tendon.

Now let's take a closer look at each section of the foot and the specific gland, organ, and body part to which each refers.

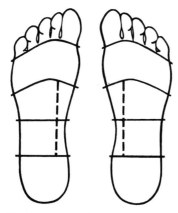

The large tendon in the arch of the foot.

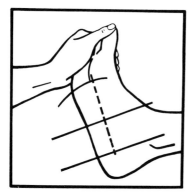

To locate the tendon, pull the toes back.

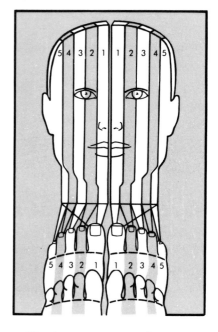

The toes correspond to zones in the head and neck.

THE TOES

The toes correspond to the head and the neck. Specifically, each big toe is the "master toe" for that side of the body because all five zones which run down that side of the body converge in this toe. Each big toe contains reflex points for the pituitary, pineal, hypothalamus, brain, temples, upper and lower jaw, gums, teeth, throat, thyroid/parathyroid, and the seven cervical (neck) vertebra.

Pituitary

Considered the master gland, the pituitary is located at the base of the brain and directly secretes or controls the secretion of almost every hormone in the body. The pituitary affects growth, sexual development, fever, fainting, pregnancy, lactation, metabolism, mineral and sugar contents of the blood, fluid retention, and energy levels—to name just a few of its activities. Its reflex point is the center of the big toe on both feet.

Pineal

A poorly understood gland in the brain that responds to levels of daylight perceived through the eye with release of the hormone melatonin. The pineal is thought to play a part in mood and circadian rhythms. It is often referred to as our intuitive gland or "third eye." Its reflex point is located in zone 1, at the inner side and top of the big toe on both feet.

Hypothalamus

This gland regulates the autonomic nervous system and controls emotional reactions, appetite, and body temperature. It has the same reflex point as the pineal.

Thyroid

Located in the neck, the thyroid controls metabolism. Its hormones regulate protein building by the body's cells, the rate at which nutrients are used by the body, and calcium levels. Metabolism affects the pace of our lives and our energy levels. The thyroid's reflex area is at the base of the big toe on both feet.

Parathyroids

Situated around the thyroid, the parathyroid glands affect calcium and phosphorus levels, which are important for muscle tone and functioning.

Seven Cervicals

The seventh cervical vertebra is the last vertebra in the neck. It protrudes at the base of the neck and can be easily felt. Many of the nerves of the arm and hand and the muscles of the neck pass by the seventh cervical vertebra. Its reflex point is located at the base of the big toe on the medial side of both feet in zone 1. The reflex points of cervicals 1 to 6 run from the base of the toenail to the seventh cervical, zone 1.

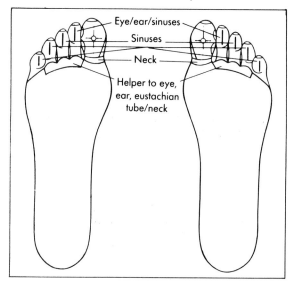

Use the small toes for fine-tuning the head and neck.

The small toes each contain one zone and are used for fine-tuning for head and neck ailments, such as sinusitis, eyestrain, hearing problems, jaw problems, and neck tension. The tips of all the toes should be worked for people with head or brain injuries and strokes.

The ridge at the base of the toes (actually on the ball of the foot) is worked as a helper reflex area for eye, ear, and eustachian tube disorders. This ridge corresponds to the neck/shoulder line; it is here that many people hold tension that can block circulation to the head.

THE BALL OF THE FOOT

The ball of the foot corresponds to the area of the body between the diaphragm and neck. Here are several vital reflex areas, including those for the heart and lungs.

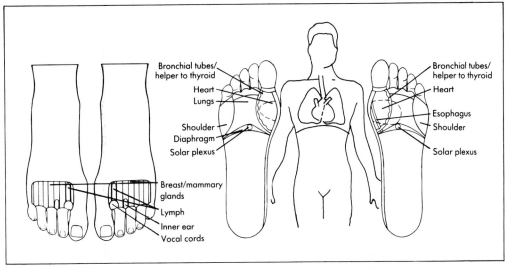

Organs, glands, and parts of the body represented on the ball of the foot.

Heart and Lungs

The *lungs* are light and spongy organs in the chest where the actual exchange of new, oxygenated air and used, deoxygenated air takes place. The *heart* is a hollow muscle which rhythmically contracts to pump the blood through the vessels in all parts of the body. Its reflex areas are on the left foot, zones 1 to 4, and on the right foot, zones 1 and 2. The chest area also contains other important structures, such as the major vessels leading to and from the heart (venae cavae, aorta), the tubes of the respiratory and digestive system (trachea and esophagus), and the nerve which controls the diaphragm.

Solar Plexus

Another important structure in this region is the *solar plexus,* or the network of nerves in the autonomic (or involuntary) nervous system which regulates the functioning of the organs. The solar plexus is located between zones 2 and 3 on both feet beneath the diaphragm line.

Lymph System

On the front of the foot, between the first and second toes, is the reflex area for the drainage of the lymphatics in the neck/chest region of the body. The lymph system parallels the network of veins in the body, and serves two important functions: to remove large proteins from the tissue and return them to circulation for eventual elimination, and to produce the cells which defend the body from foreign bacteria and viruses. The lymph system also removes excess fluid which has accumulated in tissue spaces.

THE ARCH AND HEEL

Note on the illustration how the arch of the foot is divided into two parts. The upper part corresponds to the area from the diaphragm down to the waistline. The lower part corresponds to the body from the waistline to the pelvic line.

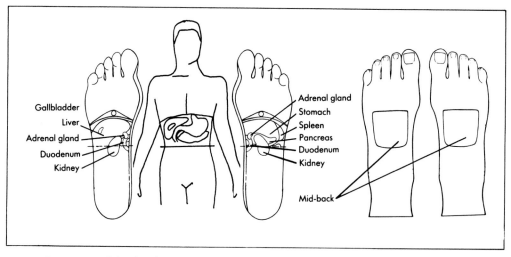

The parts of the body represented on the upper part of the arch.

The upper part of the arch contains reflex areas for the liver and gallbladder, stomach, pancreas, duodenum, spleen, adrenals, and top part of the kidneys.

Liver

The liver is the largest organ and gland in the body, located beneath the diaphragm under the rib cage on mostly the right side. Its reflex area is on the right foot, zones 1 to 5, between the diaphragm line and the waistline.

The liver processes all the nutrients from the blood, storing fats, sugars, and proteins until the body needs them. It detoxifies the blood and manufactures bile for fat digestion and important blood proteins. The liver has over 500 functions.

Gallbladder

Embedded in the liver, the gallbladder stores bile used for breaking down fats. Its reflex point is between zones 4 and 5, about two fingers above the waistline on the right foot.

Stomach

The stomach is located mostly on the left side of the body under the diaphragm. It churns food and begins protein breakdown. Its reflex area is found mostly on the left foot, zones 1 to 4, and on the right foot in zones 1 to 2.

Pancreas

The pancreas is behind the stomach, mostly on the left side of the body. Its reflex area is located mostly on the left foot, zones 1 to 4, and a little on the right, zones 1 to 1½. The pancreas controls glucose levels in the blood and is involved in the building of proteins by the cells. The pancreas also sends important digestive enzymes into the small intestine.

Duodenum

The duodenum is the first C-shaped part of the small intestine and is responsible for the breakdown of food. The average length is about ten inches. It connects the pylorus of the stomach to the jejunum. It receives hepatic and pancreatic secretions. The reflex area to the duodenum is located on both feet, zone 1, medial to the tendon, on the waistline.

Spleen

The spleen is on the left side of the body under the diaphragm and behind the stomach. Part of the lymphatic system, it produces lymphocytes and stores or filters out old and damaged blood cells. It filters the lymph of toxins and bacteria, and produces antibodies. It is an important part of our immune system. Its reflex point is found on the left foot between zones 4 and 5, about two finger widths above the waist line.

Adrenals

The adrenal glands sit on top of the kidneys and have over fifty functions. Their reflex points are on both feet midway between the diaphragm line and waist line, in zone 1. The adrenals promote normal metabolism by controlling energy levels—especially by increasing energy in response to stress. The adrenals produce cortisone and cortisol, which have anti-inflammatory properties. The adrenals may be involved in sexual development. To a large extent, the adrenals are responsible for the organ changes in fight-or-flight reactions to stress, including increased heart rate, vasoconstriction, increased breathing rate, increased efficiency of muscle contractions, and improved balance of metabolism.

The lower part of the arch contains reflex areas and points for the kidneys, ureters, bladder, small intestines, ileocecal valve, colon, and appendix.

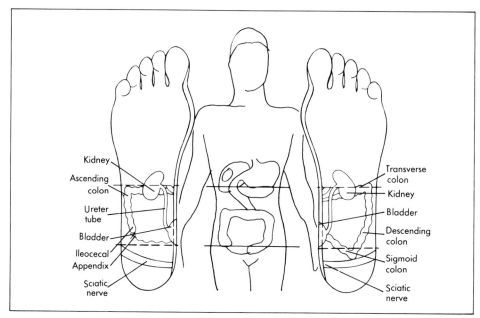

The parts of the body represented on the lower part of the arch.

Kidneys

The kidneys, in the mid-back area, are the master filters of the body. They filter toxins from the blood and produce urine. They also regulate retention of important minerals and water. Their reflex areas are found on both feet in zone 3, on the waist line.

Ureters

These tubes connecting the kidneys and bladder are passageways for urine. Their reflex areas are on both feet, in zone 1, between the pelvic and waist lines.

Bladder

The bladder, in the center of the lower abdomen, is a storage place for urine. Its reflex area is at the heel line on both feet, zone 1.

Small Intestine

The small intestine secretes some digestive juices and absorbs digested foods, water, vitamins, and minerals. Its reflex area is found on both feet from the waist line to the pelvic line inside the large intestine area, zones 1 to 4.

Ileocecal Valve

The ileocecal valve lies between the small and large intestines, prevents back-flow of fecal matter from large to small intestine, and controls mucous secretion. Its reflex point is found on the right foot in zone 5, about two finger widths below the waist line.

Colon

The colon ascends from the ileocecal valve, between zones 4 and 5, turns under the liver, crosses over at the waist line, and turns down under the spleen, to become the sigmoid colon. It absorbs water, and stores and eliminates mucus and waste material.

Appendix

The appendix, located at the beginning of the colon, lubricates the large intestine, and may secrete antibodies. Its reflex point is located on the right foot, zone 5, two finger widths below the waist line (same place as ileocecal valve).

Sigmoid Colon

This S-shaped section of the colon is the last intestinal turn before the body wastes empty into the rectum for elimination. Gas can become trapped here. Its reflex point is on the left foot, in zone 3½ at the middle of the heel.

Sciatic Nerve

Beneath the sigmoid colon and on both heels is the sciatic nerve. This is the only area that is not a reflex area but an actual nerve, running from the base of the heel up the leg and into the buttocks.

THE INNER FOOT

Look down at your feet, and notice that the inside of each foot is naturally curved to correspond to the spine. In zone 1, the area from the base of the big toenail to the base of the toe corresponds to the cervical vertebrae found in the neck. The large bulge beneath the big toe corresponds to the thoracic section of the spine (shoulders to waistline). The indentation between the middle of the foot and the heel (waist line to pelvic line) corresponds to the lumbar region. The area from the heel line to the base of the heel corresponds to the sacrum/coccyx, the very base of the spine. The reflex area for the bladder is found just below the lumbar region on the inside of each foot.

The area for the spine runs
along the inner foot.

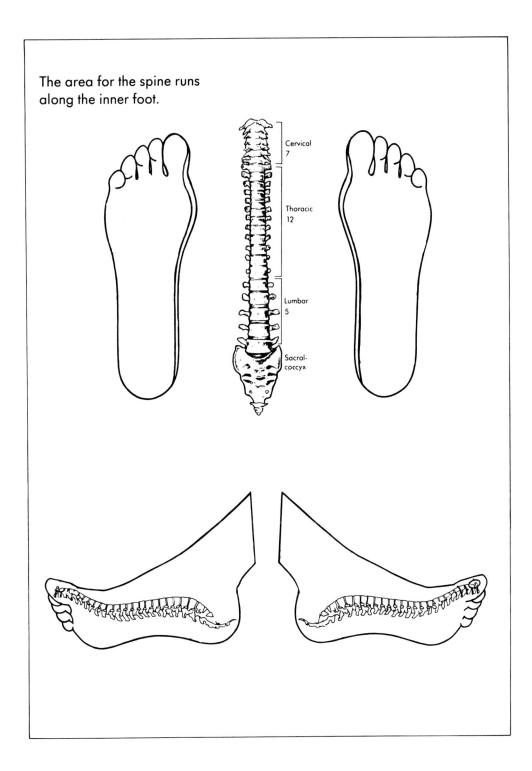

THE OUTER FOOT

Looking down at your feet, you can see that the outer edge of zone 5 corresponds to the outer part of the body: shoulder and upper arm (base of toe to diaphragm line); elbow, forearm, wrist, and hand (diaphragm line to waist line); leg, knee, and hip (from the fifth metatarsal to the heel line). (The metatarsals are the bones that run from the base of the toes down the foot to the waist line. The fifth metatarsal is easily found by running your finger down the outside of the foot to where you feel a bone sticking out on zone 5— on the outside edge of the foot at the waist line.

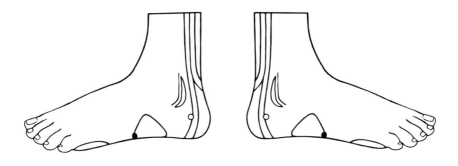

Areas of the body represented around the foot and ankle appear in the color charts.

ANKLE AREA

The area around each ankle on each foot corresponds to the pelvic area and reproductive organs. The outer ankle area contains the ovary/testicle reflex points; the inner ankle contains reflex points for the uterus/prostate, vagina, penis, and bladder. Reflex points for the fallopian tubes, lymph drainage area in the groin, vas deferens, and seminal vesicles are found in a narrow band running from below the anklebone across the top of the foot from one anklebone to the other. (See illustration.) The general chronic pelvic/rectum/prostate/uterus and sciatic nerve area begins about six inches above the anklebone and runs down to the uterus/prostate point below the ankle.

The sciatic nerve travels down both sides of the leg and across the heel like a stirrup. This is the actual nerve, not a reflex area. Therefore it is usually quite sensitive.

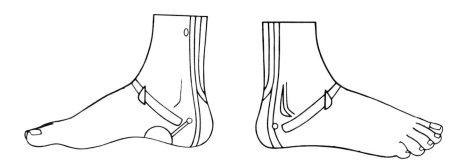

Areas of the body represented around the ankle.

Ovaries

The ovaries lie to the right and left of the uterus and produce ova and female hormones, including estrogen and progesterone, which are responsible for female sexual development. Their reflex points are located on both feet, on the outside of the ankles, midway on a diagonal from the base of the heel to the anklebone.

Testicles

These are the two glands in the scrotum that produce sperm and the male hormone testosterone. Their reflex points are found on both feet on the outside of the ankles, midway on a diagonal from the base of the heel to the anklebone.

Prostate

This gland surrounds the neck of the bladder in the male, and secretes the fluid part of the semen. Reflex points are located on both feet, on the inside of the ankles, midway on a diagonal from the base of the heel to the anklebone.

Uterus

Located in the mid-pelvic area, the uterus contains and nourishes the fetus during pregnancy. Reflex points are located on both feet on the inside of the ankles, midway on a diagonal from the base of the heel to the anklebone.

Fallopian Tubes

A pair of tubes that serve as passageways for the egg as it travels from the ovary to the uterus. Reflex areas are located on both feet across the top of the foot from one anklebone to the other.

Seminal Vesicles/Vas Deferens

The seminal vesicles are organs lying next to the prostate which store semen. The vas deferens is the tube that carries the sperm from the prostate to the urethra. The reflex areas are located on both feet across the top of the foot from one anklebone to the other.

You will learn more about these areas and how the glands and organs of the body function and how they unite to form systems as you read along. In the next chapter we'll learn the various thumb and finger techniques for working the foot and how to apply them to the different areas of the feet, and then you'll be ready to put it all together and give a full reflexology session.

A SPECIAL WORD ABOUT REFERRAL AREAS

If the foot or leg itself is injured, you will have to work *referral areas* on the shoulder, arm and hand on the same side of the body. These are the points and energy zones that have a special correspondence to those on the legs and feet. If we were still walking on all fours as our evolutionary ancestors did, we would be more aware of the similarities; but since we walk upright and use our hands and arms in a different manner than our feet and legs, we forget that they have the same anatomical roots.

Here are the correspondences (check the diagram on page 28).

FOOT	=	Hand
SOLE OF FOOT	=	Palm of hand
TOP OF FOOT	=	Back of hand
BIG TOE	=	Thumb
SMALL TOES	=	Fingers
ANKLE	=	Wrist
CALF	=	Forearm (inner)
SHIN	=	Forearm (outer)
KNEE	=	Elbow
THIGH	=	Upper arm
HIP	=	Shoulder

When the feet are injured or too sore to be worked on directly, work the hands instead. The energy zones that run from the feet up the legs to the head have their corresponding routes running from the fingertips up the arms and shoulders. Even if your feet are not too sensitive to work on, you can still work your hands during the course of a day to enhance recovery or to work on a specific area that needs attention.

Use referral areas when the feet are swollen or too sensitive to work on. This is especially true of swelling caused by an injury. Swelling is nature's cast, surrounding and protecting the injured area. It is part of the healing process, but excess swelling—that is, swelling that persists too long—can cause adhesions in the injured area, or atrophy. Reflexology can facilitate the healing process when done either on a referral area, in the case of a foot or leg injury, or on the feet themselves, when the injury is elsewhere on the body.

I once worked on a woman who had a painful bunion on her left foot which, according to the podiatrist with whom I was associated at the time, was causing her severe headaches. The large toe is the reflex area for the head, so it made sense. Reflexology relieved her headaches but, of course, did not change the bunion structurally. Eventually the podiatrist operated. During the recovery period, I worked in the referral area on the hand which corresponds to the toe, i.e., the thumb. These sessions helped the foot to heal. Later, when the foot was better, working on the foot itself helped to break up scar tissue and restore the skin to normal.

CHAPTER TWO

LEARNING REFLEXOLOGY

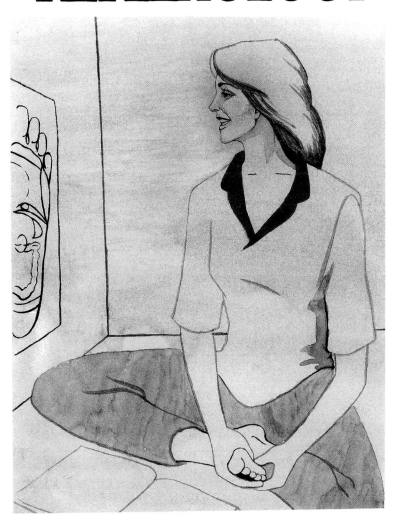

Learning the basics of reflexology is easy and fun. The foot is not mysterious, and you've been using your hands and fingers for years. Putting it all together is just a matter of learning to think about the relationship between the feet and hands in a new way and perfecting the techniques so that you become skillful in performing them. The important thing to keep in mind is that we are all natural feelers and touchers. Learning reflexology is really learning to perfect the healing skills and abilities that we were born with but have forgotten over the years or have never put into practice before.

RELAXATION TECHNIQUES

The first techniques are the playful ones—the relaxation techniques help to put your partner at ease and loosen yourself up so you can give the best reflexology you can. The first contact between your hands and your partner's feet is most important, for it is here that you build up trust. If this is your client's first reflexology session, he may feel vulnerable lying there wondering what you are going to do. The relaxation portion of the session will show your partner that it's going to be enjoyable and fun—for both of you. Remember, working on someone's feet comes naturally to most of us, and any initial hesitation you may feel is simply because you haven't handled another's feet before. Your partner may even be a bit ticklish at first due to the natural nervousness we often experience when trying something different for the first time. The relaxation techniques described below will get your partner over the ticklishness and make it easy for you to enjoy getting to know each pair of feet you work on. Practice each movement so you feel comfortable with it. In the next chapter you'll learn how to put these together in a full reflexology session.

I strongly encourage you to trust yourself and be creative. My students and associates make up great new techniques all the time. One of my instructors here at our center, Holly Papa, created many of the following relaxation techniques, which we integrated with Dwight Byers' and my own. These techniques will give you a structure to follow, but let go and work from your heart and you will be amazed at how well the techniques flow.

Relaxation and reflexology techniques are always done on bare feet, not through socks or stockings. Each of these techniques is performed on each foot. In a complete session, we do all the techniques on one foot before moving on to the other. I always apply a small amount of a non-greasy cream to the feet for the relaxation session. Clients find it soothing and comforting and it makes skin soft and flexible. Ideally, the cream should be gone by the time the actual reflexology work begins so that you don't slide over the points or find the feet too slippery to apply sufficient pressure to them. If the feet seem too greasy when you begin to work the reflex areas and points, apply a little powder or cornstarch to absorb the excess or wipe with a towel. When doing a complete hour session you can use most or all of the relaxation techniques. When doing a mini-session focusing on a particular area, do relaxation techniques that correspond with that part of the body.

Greeting the top of the feet.

Greeting the bottom of the feet.

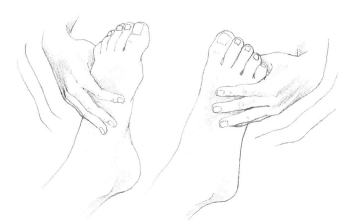

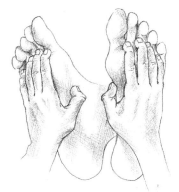

Greeting the feet: Grasp the feet and hold them in a warm, loving way. Make the initial contact by holding and pressing into them for a few minutes.

Leg stretch and lower-back release: Grasp under both feet slightly above the back of the heels, cradling the heels in the palms of your hands and supporting the ankle joints (the space between the foot and the leg). Lean backward and slowly stretch the legs out from the hip. This also stretches out the lower back. Leave the legs touching the surface that they are on. Let the weight of your body leaning backward do the work. The legs may lengthen slightly. You will notice that the leg was not fully extended from the hip joint after the person lies down. Lower-back release helps relieve tension in the lower back and hip.

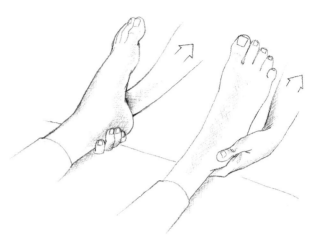

Stretching both legs and lower back release.

Ankle rocking: Rock both feet from side to side in the same direction, by holding the heels in the palms of your hands, rotating gently at the wrists, and jiggling your hands. The movement should resemble windshield wipers on a car.

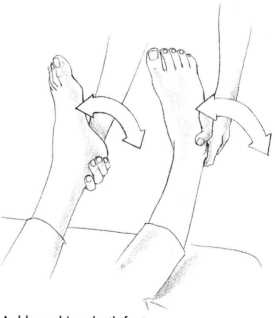

Ankle rocking, both feet.

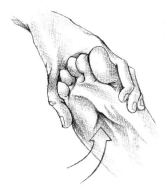

Squeeze foot to find hollow to help locate the solar plexus spot.

Thumb press: Find the hollow in the sole of the foot that corresponds to the solar plexus by placing one hand over the top of the foot at the metatarsal area and squeezing gently. The hollow that will appear on the sole of the foot at the diaphragm line is the solar plexus. You will do the thumb press on this spot. Release the foot so that it comes back to its natural shape, but remember the spot where the hollow formed. Then grasp the right foot with the left hand and the left foot with the right hand, fingers on top and thumb on the bottom so that the thumb presses on the hollow of the solar plexus point. Press the solar plexus point for a few seconds, then release, easing the pressure with the fingers first, then the thumb, but do not lose contact with the foot. Next, make gentle circular motions with the thumbs and hold the spot lightly. (Whenever transferring from one foot to the other, move the free hand to the other foot and hold the solar plexus point while continuing to hold the solar plexus point of the foot you are leaving in this way; then slowly release pressure and move on to the other foot.)

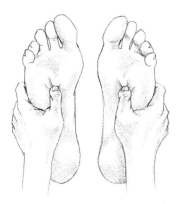

Thumb pressing on the solar plexus (two feet).

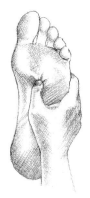

Thumb pressing on the solar plexus (one foot).

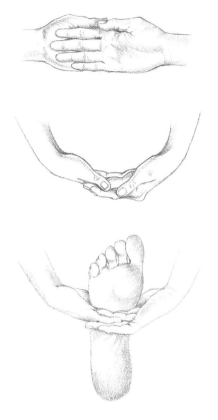

Position of the hands for finger slide.

Holding the foot with both hands for finger slide.

Index finger slide: Stand up and cradle one hand in the other so that one index finger lies on top of the other. Keeping both hands together in this fashion, hold the foot just beneath the toes so that the index fingers are on the shoulder line. The thumbs are on the top of the foot. Holding firmly, lean in with your body weight so the index fingers slide down the bottom of the foot from the neck/shoulder line to the bottom of the heel and up behind the ankles, then lightly slide back up to the toes, leaving thumbs on the top of the foot. Repeat this stroke.

Troughing—thumb slide: Stand up for a partner lying on a bed; kneel if you are on the floor. Slide the thumb down each trough between the toes on the top of the foot, applying firm pressure until you reach the diaphragm line, at which point lighten up the pressure because the skin becomes thinner and the foot bonier. Proceed down to the ankle. Trough first with one thumb, then the other so that each space receives two passes.

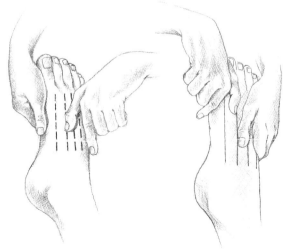

Troughing the top of the foot with the thumb (two views).

Reverse troughing with the index finger and thumb.

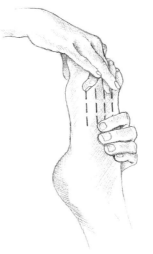

Reverse troughing: Begin at the diaphragm line, holding each trough zone between the thumb and index finger. With the index finger on the top of the foot and the thumb on the bottom, squeezing firmly, slide the index finger along the trough to where it ends between the toes.

Alternating thumb rotations: Grasp one foot with both hands so that your thumbs are on the top at the base of the toes and your fingers are supporting the foot on the bottom. Rotate one thumb at a time in small circular movements, right thumb clockwise and then left thumb counterclockwise, alternating down the foot to the ankles. Perform these same thumb rotations on the bottom of the foot, grasping the foot so that the fingers are on the top and the thumbs on the bottom. Work in small circular movements up from the heel to the toes.

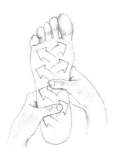

Alternating thumb rotations on the top of the foot.

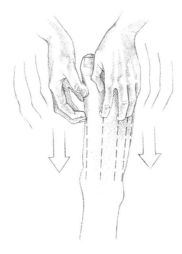

Vibrating: Run the fingertips of both hands from the base of the toes to the ankles on the top of the foot, applying firm pressure in a vibratory manner. Repeat three or four times.

One-leg rocking: Must be done on a flat, firm surface. Holding the heel in the palm of your hand, rock the foot from side to side and rotate gently at the wrist while jiggling your hand.

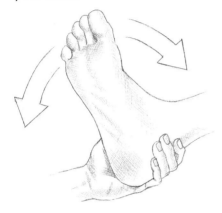

Ankle rocking one leg.

Leg bounce: Must be done on a flat, firm surface. Stretch one leg at a time, as in one-leg stretch. Then hold slightly above the heel and support the ankle joint in one hand. Place the other hand on top of the foot with the thumb pointing down toward the ankle. Now lean back slightly to utilize your body weight and bounce the leg so that the thigh muscles are bouncing on the flat surface.

One-leg stretch: Must be done on a flat, firm surface (not on pillows). Place one hand under the heel and support the ankle joint. Place the other hand across the top of the foot.
Stretch the heel toward you. Keep the foot and leg down on the flat surface.

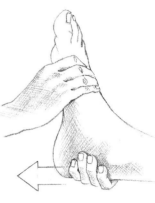

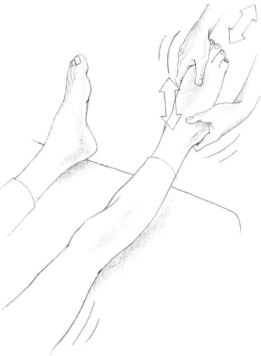

Stretching and bouncing the leg.

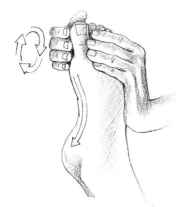

Fingertip rotations down the inside of the foot.

Fingertip rotations: With the fingertips of one hand held together, rub the inside of the foot along the spinal line in small circular patterns moving clockwise while the other hand holds the foot steady. Begin on the spinal line at the base of the big toe and work your way down to the ankle. Then proceed up the Achilles tendon and around the anklebone. Repeat this motion down the outside of the foot. (You will want to hold the foot steady with the other hand as you go down the outside of the foot. However, when you get to the anklebone, the supporting hand can make the small circular movements around the other side of the ankle, which in effect will provide the same support.)

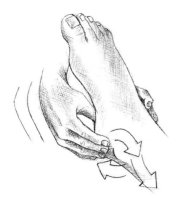

Fingertip rotations around the inside anklebone and up the Achilles tendon.

Fingertip rotations around both ankle bones and up both sides of the Achilles tendon.

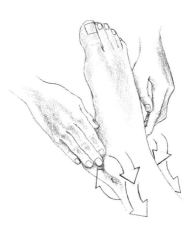

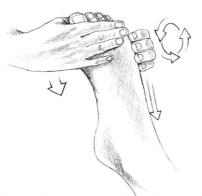

Fingertip rotations down the outside of the foot.

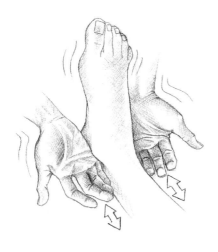

Ankle boogie: Position the hands, palms turned up, so that the fleshy area below the pinkie lies beneath each anklebone. Move the hands rapidly forward and backward in opposition to each other in a firm sawing motion, keeping the hands hooked beneath the anklebones. Maintain continual contact between your hands and the foot so that you do not irritate your partner's skin. The foot should shake from side to side when done properly.

Palm rubdown: From the position in the ankle boogie, raise your elbows and roll the palms face down and continue this back-and-forth movement, but this time with the fleshy part of the hands beneath the thumbs. You can let the thumbs themselves work the top of the groin reflex area. Rub the palms quite vigorously face down all over the foot.

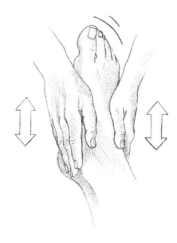

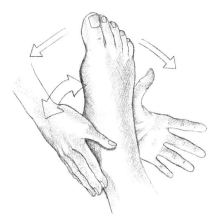 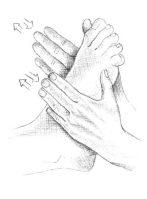

Foot boogie: Let the foot lie on the table and place one hand on each side of it. Flop the foot from side to side by lightly slapping it back and forth between your hands in a loose, flowing motion. You can also achieve the same effect by moving your hands forward and backward in a sawing motion along the edges of the foot. As one hand moves forward, the other pulls backward and so forth. The effect is similar to that of gently slapping the foot back and forth from hand to hand with the outside hand doing most of the slapping, the inside hand providing support.

Five-Toe Rotation:

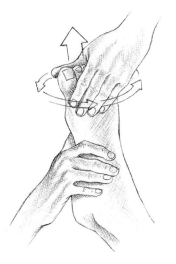

Stretch and rotate all the toes at once. Place thumb of leverage hand on solar plexus for support; fingers rest on top of foot. The working hand will stretch and rotate all toes at once.

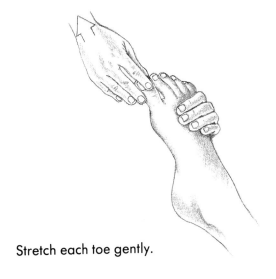

Stretch each toe gently.

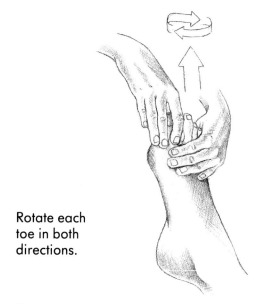

Rotate each toe in both directions.

Toe boogie: Fit the fleshy area below your pinkie between the big toe and the second toe. With the other hand positioned parallel to the first but on the outside of the big toe, rub the toe between the palms of your hands with a sawing motion. Push down firmly with the first hand to apply pressure on the webbing between the toes (for some people this area is sensitive; if so, don't apply pressure to the webbing). Use your pinkies to relax the other toes in the same manner, working up and down each toe with the hands moving back and forth in opposite directions.

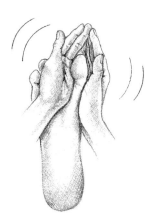

Toe stretch: Grasp each toe in turn with the thumb and index finger. Pull the toe gently out, as if you were stretching it, loosening up the joints.

Toe stretch and rotation: Gently but firmly grasp the base of each toe individually between the thumb and index finger, as for the toe stretch, and rotate it clockwise and counterclockwise.

Under-the-ankle rotations: Hold the foot slightly above the heel, supporting the ankle joint in the palm of one hand. With the other hand grasp the foot so that the heel of the hand presses into the ball of the foot (the metatarsals) and the fingers curl over the tops of the toes. Then, with this hand, rotate the foot so that it pivots on the heel held firmly by the first hand at the ankle. Stretch heel toward you as you rotate the foot. Rotate the foot in complete circles in both directions.

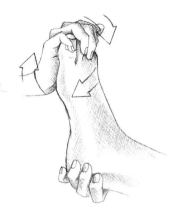

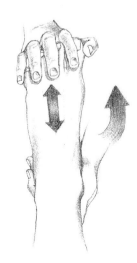

Achilles tendon stretch: Cradle the heel of one foot so that it rests in the palm of the hand. With the heel of the other hand, press forward on the ball of the foot and pull the heel toward yourself so that the bottom of the foot stretches out.

Over-the-ankle rotations: A variation on this movement is to put the hand over the top of the foot so that the webbing between the thumb and index finger fits snugly across the top of the ankle joint and the other three fingers support the foot below the anklebones. The other hand grasps the toes and rotates the foot several times in both directions as described above. This procedure stimulates the reflex points for the groin and reproductive areas and can be done in place of thumb or finger walking if this area is swollen or sensitive.

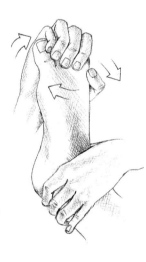

Spinal twist:

Stand up if your partner is lying on a bed; kneel if your partner is lying on the floor. With the hand closest to the leg hold the foot stationary at the arch of the foot as close to the anklebone as possible. The webbing of your hand should be on the inside edge of the foot. Place the second hand on the foot beside the first, in a similar manner keeping the index fingers next to each other on top of the foot and the thumbs next to each other under the foot. Twist gently back and forth with the second hand (the one closer to the toes). The higher hand holding the foot stationary does not move when the other hand twists. Keep your arms straight and elbows locked for better pressure. Repeat several times and then move both hands (still touching each other as described above) toward the toes, repeating as necessary until you have "twisted" the entire foot up to the base of the toes.

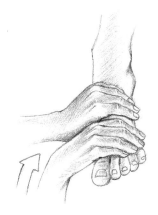

Position of hands for the spinal twist.

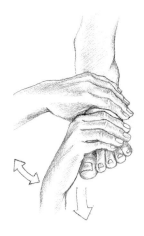

Twist the hand closer to the toes.

Lung press: Grasp the top of the foot just beneath the toes with one hand and make a fist with the other. Press the back of the fingers of the fist (not the knuckles) into the fleshy area on the ball of the foot (which corresponds to the lungs and chest). As you release the press, but still maintaining contact, gently squeeze the top of the foot below the toes (do not squeeze the toes themselves) with the other hand. Keep both hands in place on the foot even in the release. Do this several times. Alternately press, then release and squeeze in a rhythmic movement.

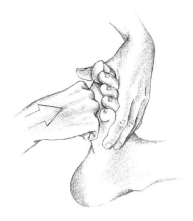

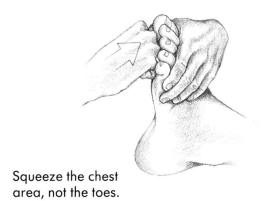

Squeeze the chest area, not the toes.

Fist slide: Hold the foot with both hands as if preparing to do the lung press. Then slide the fist down the bottom of the foot so that the backs of the fingers (not the knuckles) press firmly into the foot. Move the supporting hand under the heel as you proceed downward.

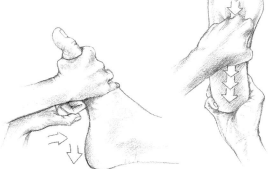

Beginning the fist slide.

Completing the fist slide with supporting hand beneath heel.

Cross thumb slide: Hold the foot with both hands so that the thumbs are on the bottom, the fingers on top for support. The thumbs should be near the sides of the foot. Press in firmly with the thumbs and let them slide toward and past each other. Then pull the thumbs back toward the edges of the foot. Work the entire sole of the foot in this manner.

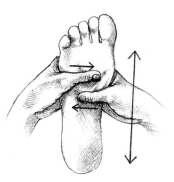

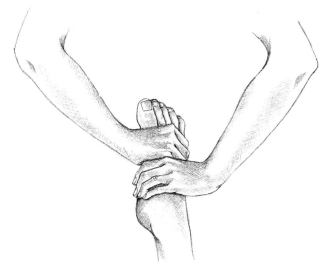

Wringing the foot: closed, tight position.

Wringing: This is similar to the spinal twist except both hands move in the wringing motion. Grab the foot in both hands as you would a wet towel and wring gently, each hand twisting in opposite directions. Your elbows should fly up and down as you do this. Move the hands gradually up the foot to "wring" the entire foot.

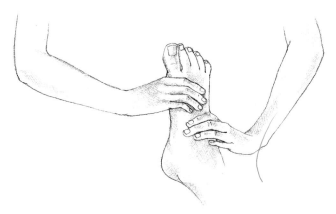

Wringing the foot: open, loose position.

Slapping: Slap the back of the hand against the sole of the foot. Slap the top of the foot with the palm.

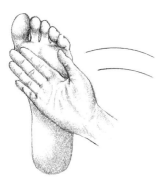

Karate chops: With the side of your hand give friendly karate chops up and down the bottom of the foot and around the heel.

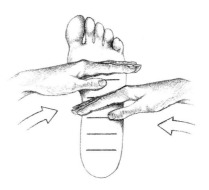

Punching: With the back of your fist, punch the bottom of the foot. Use the flat back of the hand, not the fingers or knuckles.

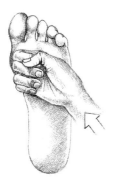

Breeze strokes: Here is the "antidote" to the karate chops. Lightly run your fingertips down the tops and bottoms and sides of each foot from the ankles to the toes in a feathery, whispy motion, barely touching the skin. Repeat several times. This procedure is very soothing to the nerves.

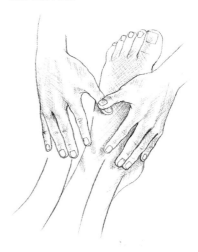

MAKE IT UP!

There are other relaxation techniques besides the ones described above. Be playful and create your own. When I teach reflexology to children I'm always amazed at how eagerly and naturally they create their own ways to relax and loosen up the feet and ankles. They pinch and punch, squeeze and slap, poke and pull. And it all works. Experiment with all these techniques and find variations of your own. As you do reflexology on your friends and family, you'll learn what each one enjoys most. Tailor your relaxation session to each person.

> There are two ways to do relaxation techniques—slowly and smoothly for deep relaxation, or vigorously for energy.

Relaxation techniques always begin and end a reflexology session, about ten minutes or so at the start and a few minutes at the close. But they can and should also be done now and then throughout the whole session. In other words, you don't need to be doing straight reflexology at all times. Whenever you feel your partner could use a little playfulness and loosening up during the session, throw in a couple of relaxation techniques and then proceed with the session.

THE BASIC REFLEXOLOGY TECHNIQUES

How to Hold the Foot

It is very important to hold the foot correctly so that the reflex points and areas are reached and stimulated properly. (See page 98 for details on positioning your partner.) You will always be holding the foot with both hands. One hand will support the foot and provide leverage for the other hand that will be doing the actual working. At times, you will want to keep the hands parallel to each other (so that both hands are holding the same section of the foot), the leverage hand on the top of the foot providing support, the working hand on the bottom. Of course, when you are working on the top of the foot, the bottom hand will provide support.

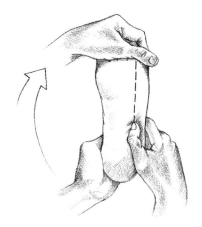

Move the holding hand from the heel to the top of the foot as the working hand progresses upward.

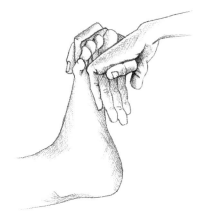

The bottom hand on the foot provides support for the hand finger-walking on the top of the foot.

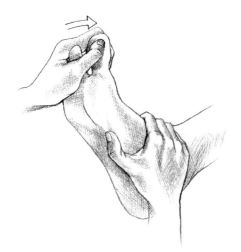

Another way to support and control the movement of the foot.

Another way to support and control the movement of the foot is to press the heel of the holding hand against the metatarsals or ball of the foot, letting the fingers curl up and over the toes. The thumb presses gently against either the big toe or the little toe, depending on the hand that you are using. Practice this hold and notice how easy it is to push the foot slightly away from you or bring it forward.

Always hold the foot firmly but gently. You may find at the start that you are reluctant to apply strong pressure to the foot (most people's feet can take more than you think!). With practice you'll learn how to be aggressive enough with your movements to provide maximum benefit without being rough or causing pain. We always work to our partner's comfort/pain threshold and not beyond. Watch body and facial language for indications of this (tightening up, jerking away, sudden deep breathing, or a long pause in the breathing pattern).

Freely switch hands as you work the foot, sometimes using one for support and working with the other, then reversing. It's important to work the reflex points in as many directions as possible, coming from the left, right, up, down, and so forth. The reason for this is that sometimes a point will be sensitive from one direction but not another. It may also be easier to reach or apply pressure with one hand than the other or from one direction than another.

Now let's learn the six key reflexology techniques, which were developed by Eunice Ingham and taught to me by Dwight Byers.

1. THUMB WALKING

Thumb walking is done with the outer edge of the thumb. To find this spot lay your hand on the table, palm downward, and notice the edge of the tip of the thumb that touches the surface. This is the part of the thumb that comes into contact with the foot. Thumb walking consists of bending the thumb at the first joint so that the thumb takes very small steps (or "bites") along the foot. Do not allow the thumb to bend at the second joint closer to the wrist. Practice taking these small bites first on the table and then on the palm of your hand or up your arm. Apply leverage with the other four fingers behind the palm or wrist and let the thumb walk along taking little steps each time it bends. It is actually the bending motion that moves the thumb forward. You don't have to consciously push it along. In other words, the little "bites" are really bites, pulling back the flesh of the skin and then moving the thumb slightly forward for the next bite. The walking movement is always forward, never backward or sideways.

At first you will probably take larger steps than is appropriate. Most people do. To refine your techniques, concentrate on taking smaller and smaller steps each time. You really cannot take steps that are too small.

Steady pressure is important. You should not feel the pressure turned on and off as your thumb walks along. There should be a steady, even pressure created as much *by the four fingers providing leverage* as by the thumb itself. Also, the position of the wrist regulates the pres-

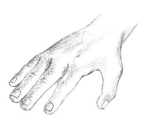

Use the outside edge of the thumb for thumb walking.

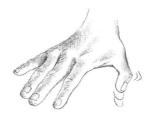

Bend your thumb at the first joint.

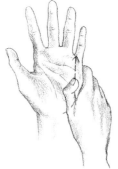

Practice thumb walking on the palm of your hand.

sure. When the wrist is raised, there is less pressure. As the wrist goes down, the pressure increases.

Thumb walking is done on the large, fleshy areas of the soles of the feet. Practice on someone. With the thumb-walking hand, place the four fingers on the top of the foot and walk the thumb up the zones in the chest area on the ball of the foot. Practice in this fleshy area until you get the knack of it. Then thumb walk up each zone along the entire length of the foot.

When you walk up the five zones on the entire foot, begin at the base of the heel, zone 5. When you reach the heel line, move the leverage hand up to the toes and gently bend them back with your thumb. This will expose the tendon in the arch so you can avoid thumb walking on top of it, and it will bring the reflex areas to the surface of the skin so you can stimulate them more easily. Reposition your leverage fingers as your hand moves forward. Keep the pressure as consistent as possible.

For working most of the foot from the heel line upward, place the heel of your holding hand against the metatarsals and gently wrap the fingers over the toes. Press the thumb against either the big toe or the little toe (depending on which hand you are using). This will give you control and permit you to push the foot backward or forward more easily.

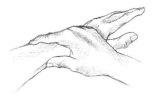

Elevate the wrist for less pressure.

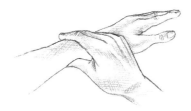

Lower the wrist for more pressure.

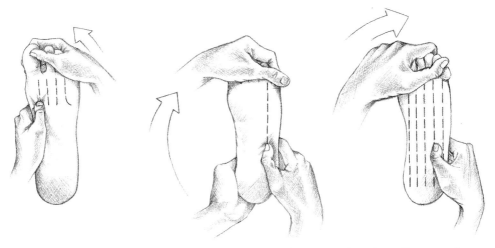

Thumb walking the chest region on the foot.

When you reach the heel line, move the leverage hand up to the toes.

Thumb walk up each zone along the entire foot.

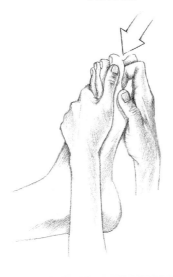

Controlling the movement of the foot.

You may notice that your hands become cramped at first because you are not accustomed to using them in this way. In a short time and with practice, you will build up the muscles required for these movements and you'll learn how to use your hands properly for leverage and support. Also, you'll know how to alternate using thumbs and fingers, and this too will make giving reflexology easier.

2. FINGER WALKING

Finger walking is similar to thumb walking except that it is the corner edge of the index finger that does the walking. Bend the finger from the first joint, keeping the rest of the finger rigid. You can give your index finger more support by holding the foot with your thumb and middle finger. Practice finger walking on the back of your hand, placing the thumb on the palm and use the other three fingers for leverage. As with thumb walking, take the smallest bites possible, slowly progressing forward; the other fingers and thumb provide leverage and move along with the index finger. It helps to raise and lower the wrist with each bite.

You can use other fingers besides the index for finger walking, and in some areas on the foot, another finger may be in better position. Usually only one finger is used at any one time, but there are places (on the sides of the foot, for example) where you can and should use two fingers for added strength.

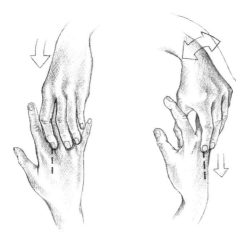

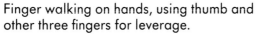

Finger walking on hands, using thumb and other three fingers for leverage.

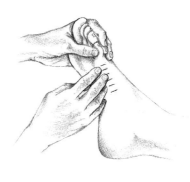

Finger walking on the side of the foot using two fingers.

Finger walking is the best technique for working the bony areas on the top of the foot and around the ankle where the flesh is thin. The fingers are not as strong as the thumbs and therefore you work more lightly in this sensitive area.

3. ROTATION ON A POINT

Press the thumb into the point you want to work; the fingers support the thumb by being opposite and parallel to it. The holding hand lifts the foot up, flexes it down and rotates the foot in a circular motion onto the thumb so it presses firmly into the point.

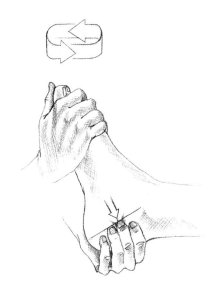

Rotating on the uterus/prostate point.

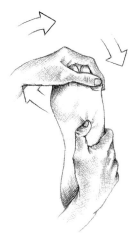

Rotating on a point.

This procedure is recommended for tender reflexes because it diverts the person's attention away from the sensitivity, whereas simple pressure alone would focus the attention directly upon it.

Always use the thumb for the rotation on a point except on the uterus/prostate point where you will use the third finger.

4. PIVOT ON A POINT

An alternative to the rotation on a point is the pivot technique. Basically, it is thumb walking while the other hand presses the foot straight back and pivots it away from you onto the thumb. To do this, grasp the foot with the holding hand, fingers resting over the top of the foot. Thumb walk with the other hand on a diagonal across the area to be worked. As you thumb walk, use the holding hand to pivot or twist the foot away from you on and off the thumb in a smooth, rhythmical fashion (only from the inside of the foot to the outside).

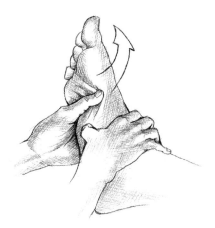

Pivoting on a point.

5. FLEXING ON A POINT

This is the same procedure as pivoting on a point, except the holding hand moves the foot backward and forward on the thumb instead of pivoting or twisting away.

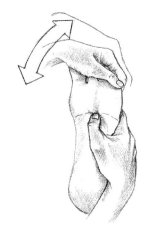

6. HOOK AND BACK-UP

This technique is used to apply pressure to a specific point that is either hard to reach deep in the foot or too small to use the walking techniques. To do it, use the four fingers for leverage, as in the thumb press (which you learned as a relaxation technique), and apply pressure with the outside edge of the thumb on the specific point. Then pull the thumb slightly backward without releasing the pressure. Do not let the thumb slide off the spot. Hold the position for a few seconds and release. Practice this on the fleshy area of your palm and in the center of the thumb or big toe.

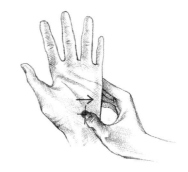

Hook and back-up.

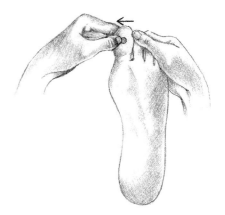

Hook and back-up on pituitary.

Hook and back-up is done on the foot for points corresponding to the pituitary, pineal, hypothalamus, the sigmoid flexure, the ileocecal valve, and the appendix.

SPECIFIC ADVICE FOR SPECIFIC PARTS OF THE FOOT

Now that you have learned the six basic techniques, let's take a look at how to apply them to various parts of the foot.

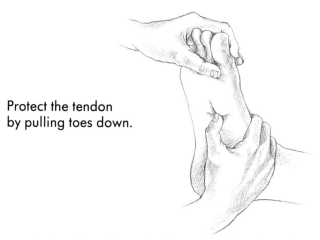

Protect the tendon by pulling toes down.

In general, thumb walk up the bottom of the foot along each zone beginning with zone 5 and proceeding to zone 1. Remember not to thumb walk up the sensitive tendon between zones 1 and 2. You can also pull the toes downward so the foot is less taut (i.e., fleshier) around the tendon. You will need to switch hands from time to time since some zones are easier to reach with one hand than the other. In fact, to be thorough, walk up each zone at least once with each hand.

HEAD AREA

(Upper third of toes: brain, pituitary, pineal, hypothalamus; middle third of toes: nose, sinus; lower third of toes: teeth, gums, jaw)

Thumb walk *down* the toes from the tip to the base of each toe, providing leverage for the thumb with the index finger. Walk all five zones in each big toe. Make three passes down each of the smaller toes: once down the center of the toe and once on each side. Take about ten to fifteen tiny bites in each pass. Change hands whenever necessary to improve access to a toe.

Thumb walk up the toes, using the thumb and fingers of the supporting hand to leverage the toes. Finger walk down the fronts of the toes, taking approximately the same number of bites and passes as you did on the undersides. Finger walk across base of fronts of toes also.

Some people's toes are permanently crooked or curled up. Be careful not to try to straighten them out completely to make it easier for you to reach them. In general, most people's toes can handle a little straightening out, but always respect the natural condition of your partner's toes.

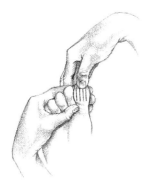

Thumb walk down the five zones of the big toe.

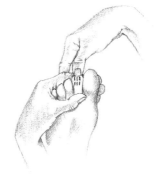

Thumb walk down the smaller toes making three passes on each.

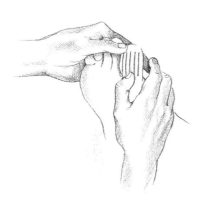

Thumb walking up the toes.

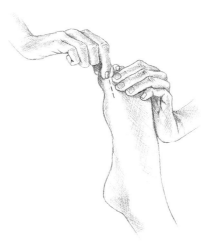

Finger walking down the fronts of the toes.

Roll the end of the index finger across the top of each toe, using the thumb and the middle finger to hold the index finger and apply pressure. This is the reflex area for stimulating the top of the head and the brain. You can also roll the tips of the toes with the flat surface of the thumbnail.

To work the pituitary gland reflex point, you must first find it in the center of the big toe. Locate the widest point on each side of the toe and draw an imaginary line from one point to the other. The line may not necessarily be horizontal; it could slant. Then draw an imaginary cross. The pituitary point is located at the midpoint of these lines.

Work the pituitary point by supporting the toe with the holding hand so that the toe doesn't bend or get pinched. Lay the fingers of the working hand over the fingers of the holding hand. Then settle the thumb slightly beyond the pituitary point, coming in from the medial side of the foot, and use the hook and back-up technique to apply pressure.

To work the points for the pineal and hypothalamus glands, work in the same way as for the pituitary, using hook and back-up on the inside edge of the big toe.

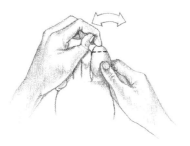

Finger rolling the top
of the toe.

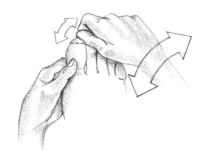

Rolling the tops of the toes
with the thumbnail.

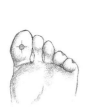

The imaginary cross to locate the pituitary gland.

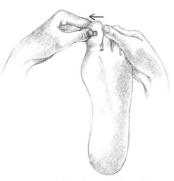

Hook and back-up on pituitary gland.

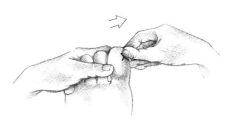

Hook and back-up on pineal and hypothalmus glands.

NECK AREA

(Neck, thyroid, parathyroid, tonsils, lower and upper jaw, helper to eyes and ears)

Thumb walk or finger walk along the neck and shoulder line (the ridge at the top of the ball of the foot). To do this, pull the pad of the foot downward with your holding hand to thin out the flesh (thumb pulling down on the bottom, fingers on the top supporting and pulling down). Always walk across the ridge from both directions, changing hands to do so. [*Note:* This is the only area where you should use the *inside* corner of

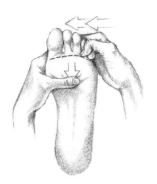

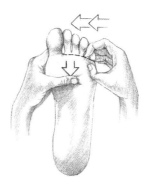

Thumb and finger walking the shoulder line.

the thumb instead of the outside corner.]

The reflex areas to the thyroid and parathyroid glands are found at the base of the big toe just above the neck line. To work this area, support the big toe with the holding hand. The fingers of the working hand rest on those of the holding hand. Thumb walk across the thyroid/parathyroid area, making at least two passes, to cover the width of this area. Change hands to walk the area from the other direction.

Work the point for the seventh cervical vertebra by steadying the big toe between the thumb and fingertips. Place the thumb of the working hand on the bottom of the foot and then finger walk around the base and across the front of the toe. Angle your finger so it fits into the groove at the base of the big toe. This is also the area for the tonsils, lower and upper jaw.

Working the ridge for the neck and shoulder line frees energy blocks to the head, and improves circulation to the eyes and ears.

An alternate way to work the neck area is called "hanging on the ridge." Press down on the ridge with the tips of the fingers to reach deep into the whole neck area. Apply firm pressure for a few seconds.

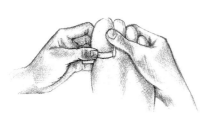

Thumb walking the thyroid and parathyroid.

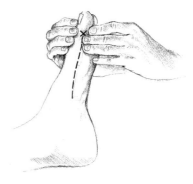

Finger walking the seventh cervical on the side of the toe.

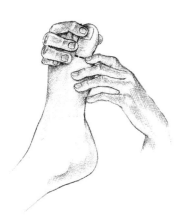

Finger walking the seventh
cervical on the front of
the toe.

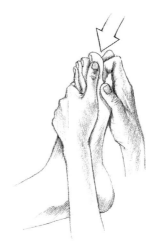

Hanging on the ridge of
the toes.

CHEST AREA

(lung, breast, heart, shoulder, esophagus, bronchial, lymph drainage,
diaphragm, helper to the thyroid, thymus)

There are five basic movements for this important area, three on the bottom
of the foot and two on the top.

1. Pull the toes back with the holding hand, the palm pressing downward
    and the fingers cupped over the top of the toes. Then thumb walk up
    the troughs extending from the space between the toes to the grooves
    between the metatarsal bones, from the diaphragm line to the shoulder
    line on the bottom of the foot. You may need to open up this area before
    you thumb walk by pushing on the ball of the foot with the heel of the
    hand. Push and spread the ball of the foot and separate the toes to bring
    the reflex areas to the surface.

2. Finger walk down the troughs on top of the foot all the way to the
    diaphragm line. It helps to spread the toes apart and press forward from
    under the foot with the fist of the holding hand when working on the

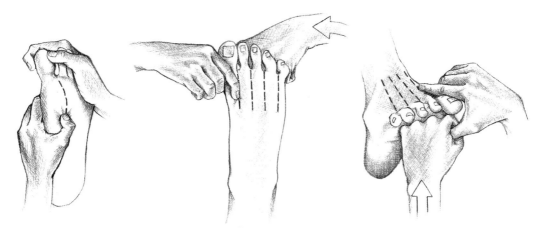

Thumb walking up the troughs between the toes.

Finger walking the chest area on the front of the foot.

Finger walking the chest area, showing the position of the thumb.

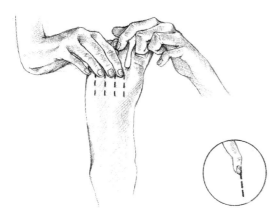

An alternate way to finger walk the chest area.

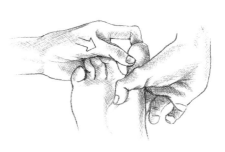

Alternate finger walking of chest area (back view).

tops of the feet to get into the troughs without hurting them. The areas for lymph drainage, whiplash, and vocal cords are in the trough on the top of the foot between the big toe and second toe.

3. Another way to finger walk down the troughs of the chest area is for the holding hand to spread two toes apart while the thumb of the working hand presses into the ball of the foot and the finger walks down the trough on top of the foot in a forward motion (not sideways).

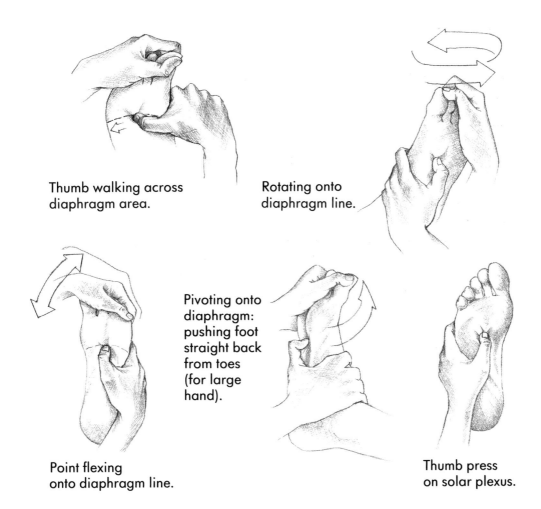

Thumb walking across
diaphragm area.

Rotating onto
diaphragm line.

Pivoting onto
diaphragm:
pushing foot
straight back
from toes
(for large
hand).

Point flexing
onto diaphragm line.

Thumb press
on solar plexus.

4. Thumb walk across the diaphragm line on the bottom of the foot from
    both directions. Then rotate, flex, or pivot across the diaphragm line.

5. Use the thumb press on the solar plexus point (which lies between the
    second and third zone where it crosses the diaphragm line). Grasp the
    foot with one hand, fingers on top and thumb on the bottom, and press
    the thumb into the point corresponding to the solar plexus. Hold it a
    few seconds, then release. You can also work the thumb in small circular
    movements in both directions over the solar plexus point. Finish off by
    simply holding the point gently with the thumb without applying pres-
    sure.

INTERNAL ORGANS AND GLANDS ABOVE THE WAISTLINE

(right foot: adrenal, liver, gallbladder, stomach, duodenum, pancreas, top of kidney; left foot: adrenal, spleen, stomach, duodenum, pancreas, top of kidney)

Look at the color charts and familiarize yourself with all the vital organs and glands whose reflex areas lie between the diaphragm line and the waist line. You will thumb walk this area. It is best to walk diagonally, hopping over the tendon when you come to it. Bend the toes backward to thin out the flesh and to open up the reflex areas. This will also expose the tendon so you can locate it, but bend the toes toward you when working near the tendon. Make several crosshatches in this large area of the arch so you cover all the points. Then reverse hands and make several passes from the other direction.

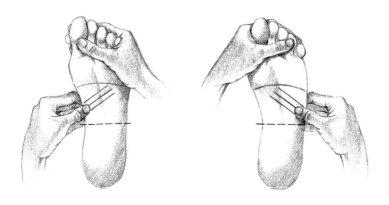

Cross hatching diagonally from the waistline area to the diaphragm from both directions.

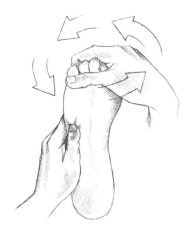

Rotating onto gallbladder point.

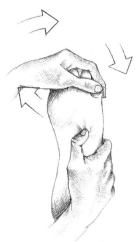

Rotating onto spleen point.

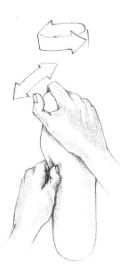

Rotating and pivoting onto adrenals point.

Rotate or pivot on the gallbladder (right foot, two finger widths above the waist line, zone 4), spleen (left foot, two finger widths above the waist line, zone 4) and adrenals (midway between diaphragm and waist lines on the medial side of the tendon, zone 1).

INTERNAL ORGANS BELOW THE WAISTLINE

(right foot: appendix, ileocecal valve, ascending colon, transverse colon, small intestine, kidney, ureter, bladder; left foot: sigmoid colon, descending colon, transverse colon, small intestine, kidney, ureter, bladder)

The reflex points for organs below the waistline are worked in the same manner as those above the waist line. On the right foot, locate the point for the ileocecal valve (two fingers below waist line in zone 5) and use the hook and back-up technique on it. Then walk up the ascending colon area in zone 5 to the fifth metatarsal bone, rotate on the hepatic flexure, and cross over at a ninety-degree angle to walk the transverse colon area, which is just below the waist line. Next make several diagonal and horizontal passes from both directions across the entire area. As before, let up the pressure when crossing the tendon. Likewise, work the heel area in all these directions.

Thumb walk the bladder point, up the reflex area for the ureter, zone 1 to the waist line. Cross the tendon beneath the waist line to the area between zones 2 and 3. Thumb walk and rotate onto the kidney point.

On the left foot, using the left thumb, begin at the bladder point. Start where the heel line intersects the inside edge of the foot and proceed downward at a forty-five-degree angle to the sigmoid flexure between zones 3 and 4. Use hook and back-up at this point. Then, thumb walk up the area for the descending colon (in zones 5 to 1) and rotate on the splenic flexure and thumb walk on a 90° angle across the area for the transverse colon (zone 5-1) below the waist line. Lastly, walk the entire area from the waist line to the bottom of the heel in several directions: vertically, horizontally, and diagonally.

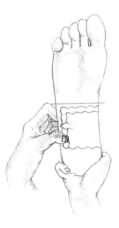

Hook and back-up on ileocecal valve and appendix.

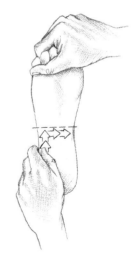

Thumb walking up ascending colon to waist line and across tranverse colon.

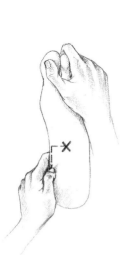

Thumb walking the bladder and ureter tubes to the kidney.

Cross hatching between pelvic line and waist line.

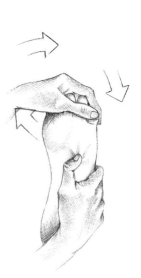

Rotating onto kidney.

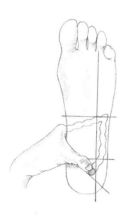

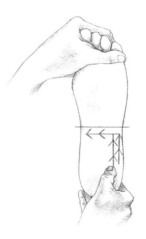

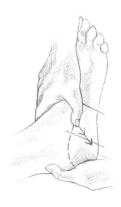

Hook and back-up
on sigmoid colon.

Thumb walking
descending colon and
transverse colon.

Alternative way to
thumb walk down from
bladder to sigmoid
colon.

An alternate way to work the sigmoid flexure is to proceed in the same way using the right thumb to come down from the bladder point. (Some people have more strength with their right hand and it is a deep point to get into.) When working the sigmoid colon, we always come from the inside of the foot towards the outside as we thumb walk down on the diagonal. We get better leverage doing it that way.

THE ARM, ELBOW, AND HAND AREAS

On the outside of the foot (zone 5) are the areas that correspond to the shoulder, arm, elbow, and hand. Hold the foot with the fingers on top of the foot for leverage. Thumb walk horizontally across the outside edge as many times as it takes to work your way from the heel line up to the shoulder line. Each run should be just a little higher than the preceding one. You should change hands as you go so that you walk the edge of the foot from both directions.

When you have finished thumb walking the entire length of the foot, finger walk it as well in the same fashion. In some ways, finger walking is more effective here because the finger can explore and work the many ridges and grooves found in this bony area of the foot.

Yet another technique is to thumb and finger walk vertically up and down the outside edge of the foot.

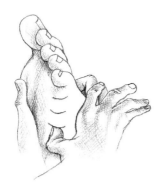

Thumb walking across outside edge of foot from pelvic line to shoulder line.

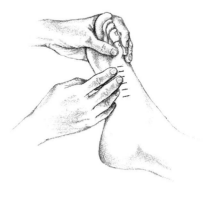

Finger walking outside edge of the foot using two fingers.

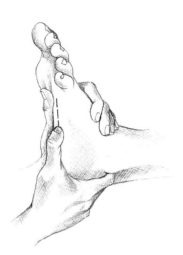

Thumb walking vertically up the outside edge of the foot.

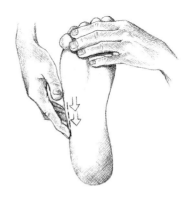

Finger walking down outside edge of foot from shoulder to base of heel.

SPINE

Tilt the foot slightly outward. Thumb walk the length of the reflex area for the spine (zone 1) from the base of the heel up to the area at the base of the toenail which is the point for the first cervical vertebra. Switch your hand position. Thumb or finger walk the seventh cervical area at the base of the big toe from several directions. Switch hands and thumb walk down the spinal reflex area, using the top of the other hand for support. Further attention can be given the spinal area by thumb walking horizontally across the edge of the foot, starting at the base of the heel and moving upward on each run as you did on the outside edge of the foot for the arm, elbow, and hand areas. Rotate and pivot onto each point corresponding to each vertebra of the spine. (There are 26 vertebrae.)

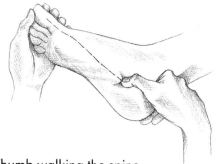

Thumb walking the spine. Notice how the fingers support under the heel when walking from base of heel to pelvic line.

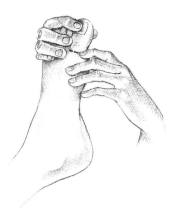

Finger walking across the seventh cervical.

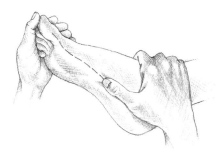

Swing fingers over ankle and move them up the foot as you thumb walk up the spine.

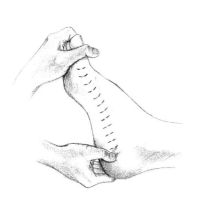

Thumb walking across the spine.

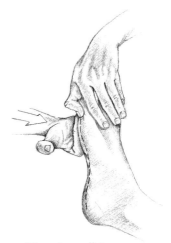

Thumb walking
down the spine.

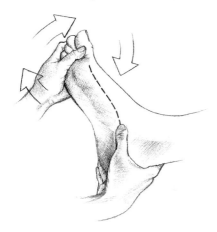

Rotate onto each vertebra
of the spine.

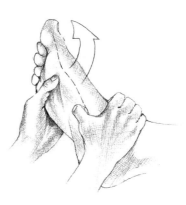

Pivot onto each vertebra
of the spine.

HIP, LEG, KNEE

There is a triangular indentation on the outside of the foot that corresponds to the leg, knee region. This area has been found to relate to the hip and lower back as well. On the outside of the foot the triangle is formed by the end of the fifth meta-tarsal bone, the front edge of the heel line, and the bony area farther up the side of the foot. As you feel around for it, you'll notice that your fingers sink in slightly since the area doesn't have the bony underpinning of the areas around it. Finger walk this area, making several passes from different directions.

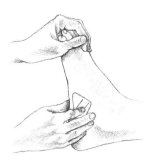

Finger walk up hip, knee, leg, lower back.

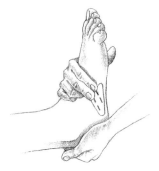

Finger walk down hip, knee, leg, lower back.

CHRONIC AREA AND SCIATIC NERVE

The area around the Achilles tendon is worked for chronic ailments related to the prostate, uterus, and rectum as well as problems with the sciatic nerve. Work this area on the inside of the right foot by holding the ball of the foot with the left hand and tipping the foot out and pushing back. Place the right hand on the top of the lower leg six inches above the anklebone, and thumb walk down the Achilles tendon area toward the heel. (This is a very sensitive area. Do not apply too much pressure.) Then thumb walk across the sciatic nerve line on the bottom of the heel, and finger walk up the outside of the foot along the Achilles tendon. Reverse hands for working on the left foot. There is another point to work for the sciatic nerve and hip found behind the outside ankle bone—shaped like a crescent moon. Gently finger walk under and up this area several times.

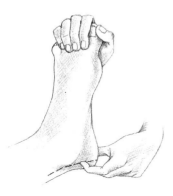

Finger walking up inside
of leg behind ankle bone
for sciatic nerve.

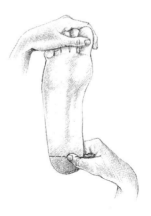

Thumb walking across
sciatic nerve.

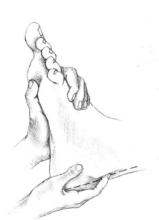

Finger walking up outside
of leg behind ankle bone
for sciatic nerve.

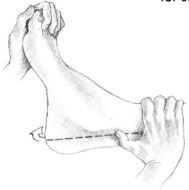

Thumb walking down
sciatic nerve.

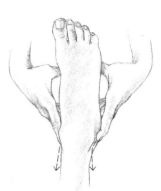

Finger walking both
sides of sciatic nerve.

HEEL AND ANKLE AREAS

Use thumb walking on the fleshy bottom part of the heel. Finger walk the areas around the ankle where the flesh is thinner. The band that runs from below the inside ankle across the top of the foot to the opposite ankle (lymph, groin, and fallopian tube and vas deferens areas) should be finger walked from both directions. It tends to be a very sensitive area, but you can thumb walk if you work gently. Rotate the thumb into hollow on top of the ankle. Do the over-the-ankle rotation.

The points for the uterus/prostate (inside of ankle) and the ovaries/testes (outside of ankle) can be found midway on a line drawn from the anklebone to the back of the heel. To locate these points exactly, put the tip of the index finger or thumb on the anklebone and the tip of the pinkie on the back corner of the heel. Then align the third finger midway between the two so that all three fingers lie in a straight line. The third finger should be resting on the point. Use this procedure on both sides of the ankle.

Work the uterus/prostate point by cupping the heel with one hand and curling the third finger so that the finger tip fits into the point. Then rotate the foot with the other hand several times in both directions as you apply pressure to the uterus/prostate point.

After locating the ovary/testicle area on the outside of each foot using the three-finger method described above, work the point and the area around it by doing small circular finger rotations and finger walking.

It will take some practice before you will feel comfortable and knowledgeable about working all these parts of the foot. Eventually it will become second nature to you. Don't be discouraged if it doesn't come as fast as you would like. Refer back to this book whenever necessary.

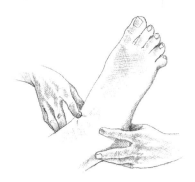

Finger walking in both directions for lymph, groin, fallopian tube, seminal vesicles area.

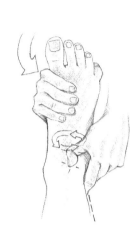

Rotating thumb into hollow at lymph/groin area.

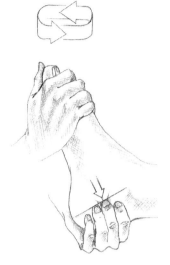

Rotate onto uterus, prostate.

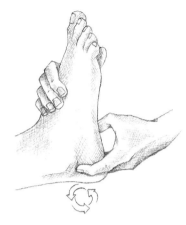

Small circular finger movements on ovaries/testes.

WHAT CLIENTS MAY EXPERIENCE

Every person you work on is unique. No two people react in exactly the same way to reflexology, nor does the same person always experience the same things each time he or she receives a treatment. When doing reflexology, therefore, it is important to be aware of the various responses that may occur in your partner.

Most people experience deep relaxation, tranquility, and serenity. Don't be surprised if someone falls asleep in the middle of a session. Sleeping is good, and reflexology works just as well whether a partner is in dreamland or consciously monitoring every move you make. When the session is over (and the sleepers wake up!), most people will say they feel more balanced, revitalized, perked up, although in the first few seconds they may feel a bit disoriented, as most of us do when waking up from a deep sleep.

Some people, however, may experience fatigue, especially if they release a lot of toxins (waste materials such as calcium deposits, excess uric acid, lactic acid, CO_2). Cleaning out the system can be exhausting, and they may report feeling rather tired afterward. Usually after the first two or three sessions, they no longer experience this fatigue. Reflexology sessions done regularly keep the system cleared, so you may find this response only from those who haven't had a session for some time.

Often people will urinate or have a bowel movement after a session. This too is part of the general stimulation and detoxification that result from reflexology.

Reflexology improves circulation and releases blocked-up energy, which can be experienced by your partner as tingling or itchiness. Sometimes the release of stress causes these sensations, which may also be accompanied by a light floating feeling. It's common for the body temperature to go down slightly when we relax. Keep a light blanket nearby in case your partner gets chilly.

Occasionally the person's foot may cramp up a bit. You can relieve the cramp by doing the breeze strokes, wringing, or slapping as you do during the relaxation session. You may need to remind your partner to keep breathing since we tend to stop breathing when we experience discomfort.

I once had a client who suffered from terrible leg and foot cramps, and nothing ever seemed to help. She traveled a lot and met with doctors all over the world and told them about her problem. Finally, a Canadian doctor, who worked with Olympic athletes, suggested that she pinch her upper lip just under her nose whenever she got a cramp. She claims that this helps to dissipate it. I have shared the remedy with many of my clients and quite a few have said it helps their cramping too.

Clients who have a lot of toxins and impurities in their system may go through what is called a "healing crisis," which can begin during the reflexology session or shortly afterward. Typical reactions in a healing crisis are headache, diarrhea, coldness, nausea, and sinus congestion. It sounds terrible, but assure your partner that the reaction is a good sign. It means the reflexology is working! It's the old story that sometimes things have to get worse before they get better. Healing crises usually pass within twenty-four hours. Because they rid the body of toxins and impurities, they are less likely to occur the next time.

GENERAL POINTERS

Now that you have learned what to do and what to expect, let's consider some general pointers about reflexology.

When giving people their first treatments, do more relaxation techniques than you would normally do. People who have never had their feet worked on before may be anxious and less flexible. They will eventually loosen up as they grow more accustomed to reflexology. Also, apply less pressure on first-timers, gradually increasing it with subsequent sessions. This slow, gentle approach should also be used in working on the elderly, small children, and the very sick.

If you discover tender reflexes on the foot (you'll know because your partner will flinch, wince, or jerk!), don't just give up on them. Instead, work to the pain threshold, then go on to other areas, and return later to work the tender area a little more. Tenderness in an area is not always a sign that something is wrong with the corresponding area in the body. It might be a foot problem such as a corn, wart, bunion, bruise, shoe irritation, scar tissue, structural problem caused by poor posture, or a hereditary defect.

It may take from five to ten sessions before you and your partner begin to see noticeable results in ongoing problems. The immediate results such as relaxation, euphoria, and serenity are almost always achieved in the earlier sessions, but don't expect chronic ailments to improve overnight. Reflexology is neither magic nor a panacea.

Medication, drugs, and alcohol reduce sensitivity. It's best for clients to abstain from nonprescription drugs and alcohol before and after a session. The clients who are on medication should stay on it, but should also inform their physicians that they are now receiving reflexology in addition to traditional medical treatment. Why? Because a relaxed body functions better and may utilize the medication more efficiently, even reaching the point where the dosage may be reduced. But only the physician can reduce it. Reflexology is not meant to replace medication, and neither you nor your partners should take it upon yourselves to make such a decision. I've discovered, though, that some of my diabetic clients, in consultation with their doctors, have been able to reduce their insulin. The same has been true for heart patients who have had their medication reduced while they stayed on a *regular* reflexology program.

When your partner asks questions during the session about what part of the body/foot you're working on, always answer in general terms. Say you are in a particular region or area, rather than working a specific organ or gland. In fact, the organs overlap on the foot just as they do in the body, and you can't always be sure which one is being worked on. Telling a partner who experiences a little tenderness in one area that you are working a specific organ or gland may be misleading or in fact wrong. So answer questions generally. For example, if you are working the chest area and your client says, "That hurts a bit" and asks what area in the body it corresponds to, don't say "the heart" or "the lungs." This may raise anxieties unnecessarily. Just say you are working the chest region.

Encourage your partner to rest during and after a session and not talk or ask questions. Try to explain as much as possible before the session begins so that he can relax. Talking uses a lot of energy. Tell your partner that if questions occur during the session, hold them and you'll answer them later.

Remember, reflexology is not used to diagnose illness. A tender area on the foot does not necessarily mean that there is trouble in the corresponding body part. Only a trained medical diagnostician can make reliable diagnoses. Lay people, however, can use reflexology to pinpoint or confirm diagnoses because the condition will be reflected in the reflex areas of the foot.

Finally, work the reflexes from several directions. Cover each area as thoroughly as possible. You cannot always be sure that you've covered specific points. Some are deep; some are quite small. By working in several directions, you stand a better chance of working all of them, and you may find that different angles will reveal tenderness or blockages that were missed coming from just one direction. Also, your techniques may be more accurate and efficient from one angle than from another.

• • •

Practice these techniques and maneuvers on yourself and your friends so that you become comfortable and skillful in doing them. Most of all, have fun with them. They are meant to be pleasurable to give and receive. You will get better the more you do them. As in learning to drive a car, there are a lot of little details to keep in mind (as well as some big ones), but eventually you'll be able to do them with your eyes closed (the reflexology, that is, not driving the car!).

In the next chapter we'll learn how to get ready for a reflexology session and how to put all these techniques together for a full treatment.

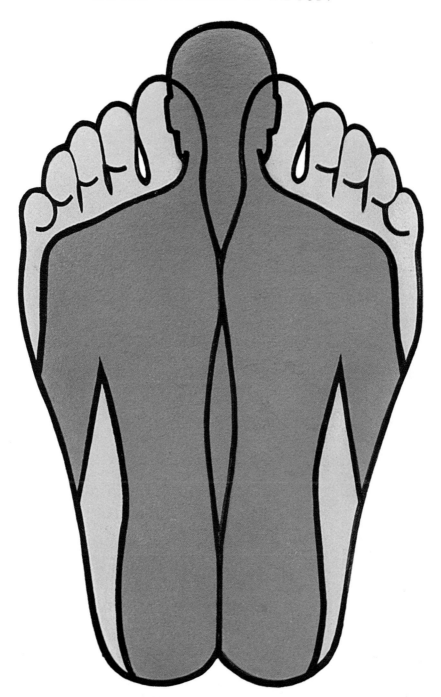

LAURA NORMAN'S FOOT REFLEXOLOGY CHARTS

1. BRAIN
2. SINUSES/OUTER EAR
3. SINUSES/INNER EAR/EYE
4. TEMPLE
5. PINEAL/HYPOTHALAMUS
6. PITUITARY
7. SIDE OF NECK
8. CERVICAL SPINE (C1–C7)
9. SHOULDER/ARM
10. NECK/HELPER TO EYE, INNER EAR, EUSTACHIAN TUBE
11. NECK/THYROID/PARATHYROID/TONSILS
12. BRONCHIAL/THYROID HELPER
13. CHEST/LUNG
14. HEART
15. ESOPHAGUS
16. THORACIC SPINE (T1–T12)
17. DIAPHRAGM
18. SOLAR PLEXUS
19. LIVER
20. GALLBLADDER
21. STOMACH
22. SPLEEN
23. ADRENALS
24. PANCREAS
25. KIDNEY
26. WAIST LINE
27. URETER TUBE
28. BLADDER
29. DUODENUM
30. SMALL INTESTINE
31. APPENDIX
32. ILEOCECAL VALVE
33. ASCENDING COLON
34. HEPATIC FLEXURE
35. TRANSVERSE COLON
36. SPLENIC FLEXURE
37. DESCENDING COLON
38. SIGMOID COLON
39. LUMBAR SPINE (L1–L5)
40. SACRAL SPINE
41. COCCYX
42. SCIATIC NERVE

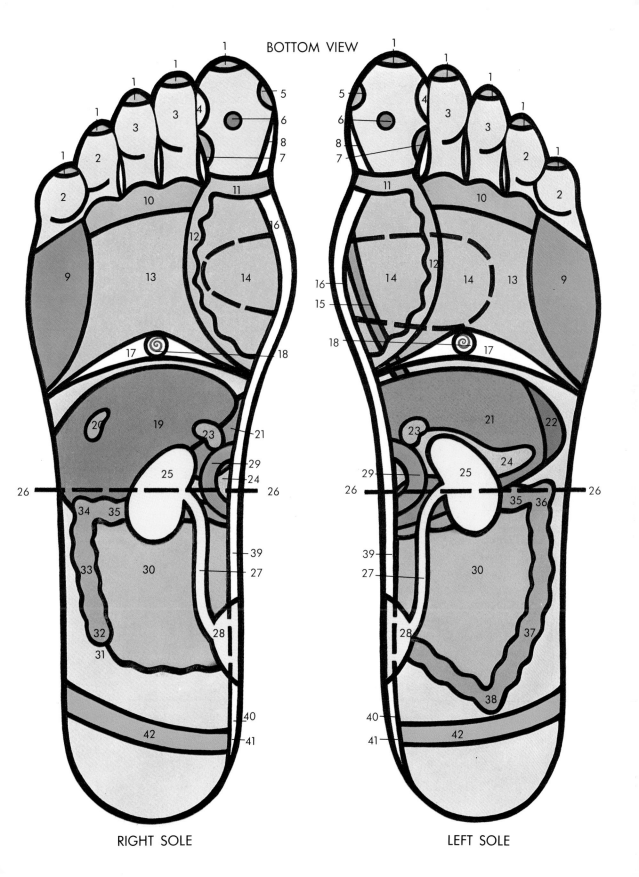

BOTTOM VIEW

RIGHT SOLE

LEFT SOLE

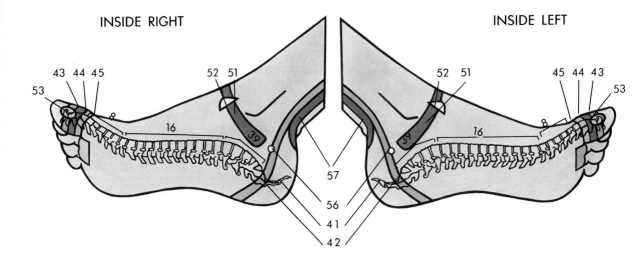

INSIDE RIGHT

INSIDE LEFT

LAURA NORMAN'S FOOT REFLEXOLOGY CHARTS

41. COCCYX
42. SCIATIC NERVE
43. UPPER JAW/TEETH/GUMS
44. LOWER JAW/TEETH/GUMS
45. NECK/THROAT/TONSILS/THYROID/PARATHYROID
46. VOCAL CORDS
47. INNER EAR HELPER
48. LYMPH BREAST/CHEST
49. CHEST/BREAST/MAMMARY GLANDS
50. MID-BACK
51. FALLOPIAN TUBES/VAS DEFERENS/SEMINAL VESICLE
52. LYMPH/GROIN
53. NOSE
56. UTERUS/PROSTATE
57. CHRONIC AREA—REPRODUCTIVE/RECTUM

TOP VIEW

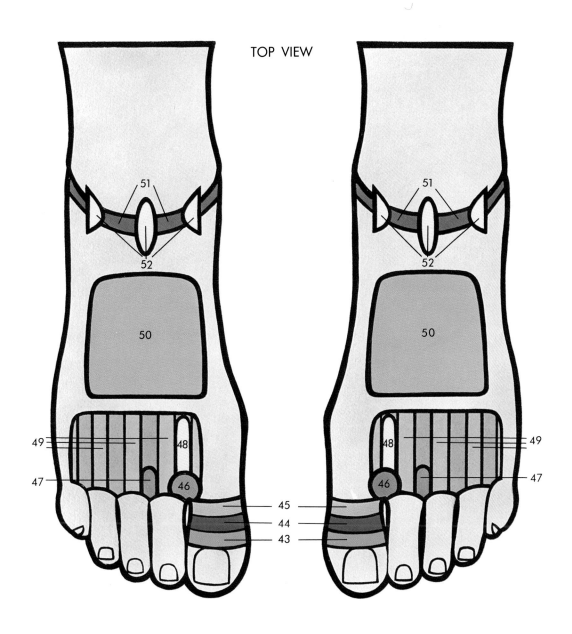

LAURA NORMAN'S FOOT REFLEXOLOGY CHARTS

LAURA NORMAN'S FOOT REFLEXOLOGY CHARTS

OUTSIDE LEFT VIEW

9. SHOULDER/ARM
42. SCIATIC NERVE
43. UPPER JAW/TEETH/GUMS
44. LOWER JAW/TEETH/GUMS
45. NECK/THROAT/TONSILS/THYROID/PARATHYROID
46. VOCAL CORDS
47. INNER EAR
48. LYMPH/BREAST/CHEST
49. CHEST/BREAST/MAMMARY GLANDS

INSIDE RIGHT VIEW

8. CERVICAL SPINE (C1–C7)
16. THORACIC SPINE (T1–T12)
28. BLADDER
39. LUMBAR SPINE (L1–L5)
40. SACRAL SPINE
41. COCCYX
53. NOSE
54. THYMUS
55. PENIS/VAGINA
56. UTERUS/PROSTATE

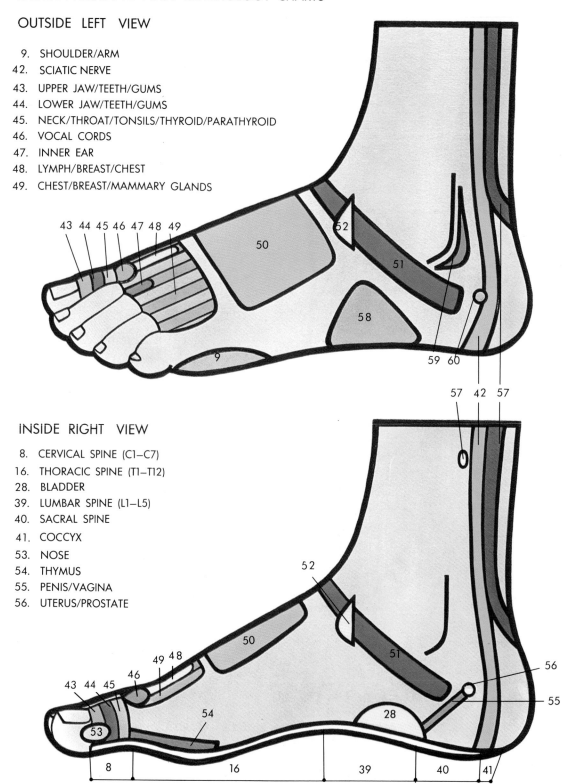

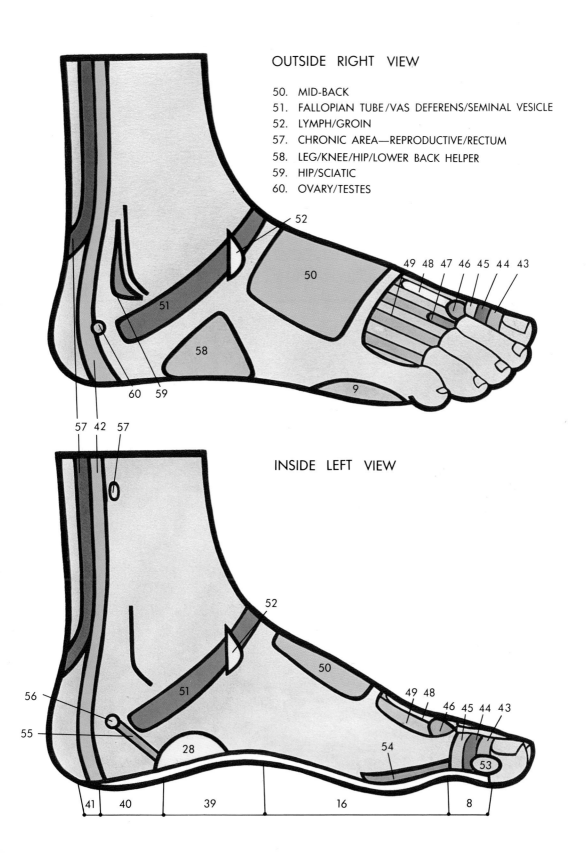

OUTSIDE RIGHT VIEW

50. MID-BACK
51. FALLOPIAN TUBE/VAS DEFERENS/SEMINAL VESICLE
52. LYMPH/GROIN
57. CHRONIC AREA—REPRODUCTIVE/RECTUM
58. LEG/KNEE/HIP/LOWER BACK HELPER
59. HIP/SCIATIC
60. OVARY/TESTES

INSIDE LEFT VIEW

LAURA NORMAN'S FOOT REFLEXOLOGY CHARTS — REFERRAL AREAS

FOOT = HAND
SOLE OF FOOT = PALM OF HAND
TOP OF FOOT = BACK OF HAND
BIG TOE = THUMB
SMALL TOES = FINGERS
ANKLE = WRIST
CALF = FOREARM (INNER)
SHIN = FOREARM (OUTER)
KNEE = ELBOW
THIGH = UPPER ARM
HIP = SHOULDER

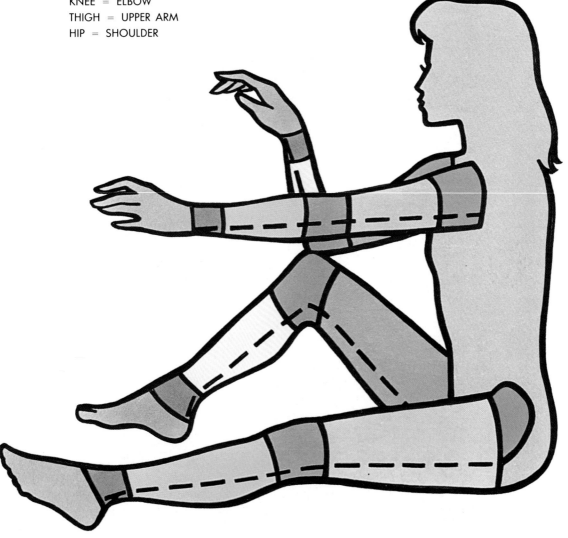

CHAPTER THREE

DOING REFLEXOLOGY

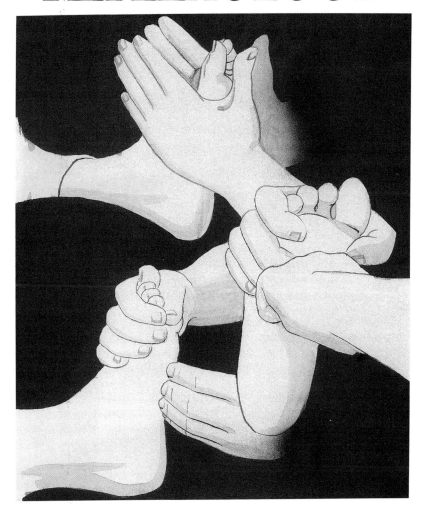

A reflexology session is much more than just working on the feet. As we've already seen, when two people come together for the benefit of one or the other, the energy circuit they create is profoundly enriching to both on physical, emotional, mental, and spiritual levels: the work itself helps the one who *gives* as well as the one who *receives*. A reflexology session is a special moment in a busy day, a time you will look forward to as much as your partner. And while it's true that spur-of-the-moment reflexology is just as beneficial as a well-planned session, you'll find that by putting a little extra care, creativity, and personal attention into your formal sessions you'll both get a lot more out of them.

Now that you've learned the principles and techniques of reflexology, let's learn how to actually "do" it—how to put into practice what you've studied and learned. We'll cover everything from getting the room ready to getting yourself and your partner ready. Then, we'll consider a typical order of treatment—how to begin, how to end, and everything in between. Keep in mind that as you become more familiar with reflexology and see the results in your own life, you'll want to personalize the way you do reflexology. You'll develop a style that is unique to you. But for now, here are some suggestions that I and my associates have developed successfully over many years and on thousands of clients.

PREPARING THE ENVIRONMENT

Reflexology does not have to be "planned"; it can happen spontaneously, anywhere, anytime, whenever the need is felt for it. But as reflexology becomes a part of your regular home life, you'll want to embellish it with rituals and a setting pleasing to the senses, one that you, your partner, family, and friends will enjoy.

First of all, choose a pleasant room in the house where you can lie down comfortably. A professional reflexologist usually uses a special "massage table," or recliner, and you may want to invest in one or the other for yourself. But it isn't necessary. A bed will work just as well. When I first began my practice sixteen years ago, I made house calls and worked on clients lying on their own beds where they were comfortable and relaxed. Simply have your partner lie down with her feet at the foot of the bed. Place a small pillow under the head to support the neck and allow you to observe facial expressions. Put a pillow under the feet if necessary to adjust the height of the feet so that, while you work on them, you are comfortable as well. Ideally, whether you are working on a bed, sofa, or table, your partner's feet should be at your chest level to minimize muscle tension in your arms and back. If you're working on a bed or couch, you'll be able to reach the feet easily by sitting on a chair, a low stool, or on the floor.

If you are used to sitting on the floor cross-legged, your partner could lie on the floor and rest her feet on a pillow in your lap. You'll want to lean against a wall or a couch to relieve any strain on your back. Experiment and be creative to find a suitable spot in your home.

If possible select a room where you can lower the lighting, close the blinds or curtains, and block outside noises. Adjust the temperature according to the season of the year so that you are both comfortable. Have a light blanket handy in case your partner gets chilly. In the cooler seasons a blanket provides that touch of warmth and coziness that makes people feel secure and free of care and worries. Take the phone off the hook, or turn on your answering machine, and tell others in the family, especially children, not to disturb you until you are finished.

Some people enjoy background music during reflexology; some want silence after too much noise and commotion at work—or even too much background music at work. Remember, the goal is to help your partner relax, so tailor the music to individual preferences, not just what you like. If music is used, choose something restful and soothing, or for a "loverly" mood, play romantic instrumental pieces. A candle and incense can also add to the atmosphere.

Many of my clients enjoy environmental tapes with natural sounds, such as waves on a seashore, birdsong, gentle breezes in the trees, night sounds, and so forth. Tapes can incorporate subliminal messages that some people find very helpful for controlling or improving other areas of personal health, such as losing weight, stopping smoking, building confidence, becoming more successful, or just plain relaxing. Playing these tapes during reflexology sessions can be very powerful because reflexology induces those deep levels of relaxation and the alpha states in which people are more receptive to suggestions.

THE IMPORTANCE OF VISUALIZATION

Along with music, your partner may want to employ visualization techniques. Although the success of reflexology is not dependent on doing so, many people discover that by using creative visualization, they relax more quickly and deeply, and ailments heal more rapidly. The value of imagery in healing has been well established in numerous studies. For anyone who wants to explore this more systematically, there are several books on the subject. But it doesn't take formal study to use visualization. We are all natural daydreamers and fantasizers. One of the remarkable findings of the many studies done with cancer patients, for example, is that almost any type of powerful, positive, healing imagery can be beneficial. It can be as bizarre or ludicrous as you want. It all seems to work.

When I worked on morning talk-show host Regis Philbin for a kidney stone, he visualized the stone slipping easily down the ureter and dissolving, even though his doctors had told him the actual stone was too large and irregularly shaped to pass of its own accord—hence their advice to undergo surgery. With the help of reflexology and Regis's own imagery, the stone passed during the night and he didn't need surgery the next morning. In later chapters, I'll recommend specific visualizations for various ailments that you can suggest to your partners.

Almost everyone can visualize to some degree. If you can close your eyes and see the face of a special person, your bedroom, or the street you grew up on when you were a child, you can visualize well enough to make visualizations a part of the healing process. Visualization, however, does not encompass only visual impressions. It also includes feelings, smells, sounds, and textures. You will want to incorporate as many sense-related impressions as you can in every visualization.

The basic guidelines for visualizing are these:

First, relax, breathe deeply (which you will already be doing if you are receiving reflexology), and clear your mind of other thoughts. Let it go blank as far as you are able.

Choose a visualization for general relaxation or one that is specific to the part of your body that needs healing. A general relaxation visualization might be to see yourself lying on a warm, sunny beach, hearing the waves, feeling the breeze blow across your body. Of course, if you are not a "beach person," this will not work for you. Choose some place either outdoors or indoors where you can relax and let go. Then visualize yourself there and try to recreate how you feel when you are there.

A visualization that is specific to a part of the body that needs healing can take several versions. You might want to imagine healing energy flowing to that part of the body and "see" it as a special color or as light. For example, if your lower back aches, you might picture a healing blue light flowing into that part of your back. You might see it first above your head and pull it into your body with each breath you inhale. Then send it to your lower back. Feel your back heal as the blue light floods that area.

Another way to work on a specific hurt or ailment is to visualize the pain or discomfort in some bold, dramatic way. Then visualize whatever it takes to counteract that image. For example, if your arm is bruised, visualize the bruise as a pool of blue-black, stagnant water that has collected in your arm. Then visualize a stream of fresh springwater flowing into it and washing the polluted waters away. Or if you have a muscle spasm, you might visualize the area in spasm as a thick rough rope tied in a hard, tense knot. Then visualize it slowly loosening up and untying. For a fever, see a blazing fire raging in your head and some helping figure throwing cold buckets of snow into the fire to put it out.

Many sores and troubles respond well by simply visualizing your own blood and energy flowing freely and easily throughout your body and especially to and through the afflicted area.

Another type of visualization is to see yourself well. Observe yourself performing the activities that will be easy for you once the affliction is gone. See yourself running, walking, dancing, making dinner, meeting a friend, or whatever will inspire you to overcome the problem. Images of ourselves as we would like to be are vehicles for getting us there. (The opposite is also true. If you think negatively about yourself or your abilities, you tend to manifest those negative qualities.)

Use visualization to the extent that it helps you during reflexology. If you find it distracting or a "chore," it would be better just to relax, clear your mind, and let peaceful thoughts come spontaneously. If you enjoy visualizing, continue it for as long as you like during the session. For visualizations to really work, you should maintain a visualization for at least two to three minutes. If you get distracted or your mind wanders, just bring it back and continue. Do it as naturally and spontaneously as you can, not straining over it. In time it will become second nature.

PREPARING FOR THE SESSION

Reflexology works best when both the giver and the receiver of the session are ready for it. Here are some specific suggestions for getting you and your partner ready physically and mentally.

First, you should know your partner's health history. Obviously you don't need to be as thorough as a medical doctor or nurse would be, but in general, ask the same type of questions regarding past illnesses, surgery, broken or injured bones, as well as current problems, any medication he may be on, and where stress is most evident in his body. You will want to focus on these areas and the related organs and glands that could be affecting these conditions. If your partner has a serious problem and has not seen a physician, encourage him to do so. Serious illnesses require a thorough evaluation and diagnosis from a reputable physician. Remind your partner that reflexology is not a substitute for traditional medical treatment, but rather an adjunct to it.

If a client is on painkillers or any medication that desensitizes feeling, I am always careful not to overwork the reflex points for the areas in question because they may be dulled due to the medication. Don't be misled into thinking that because your partner feels no discomfort when you work these areas, you can work them deeply and for greater lengths of time. In fact, just the opposite is true. Work them sensitively and for short periods of time.

Suggest that your partner abstain from stimulants such as coffee, tea, and alcohol before and after each session. The goal of reflexology is to relax, not get a buzz on! Stimulants are counterproductive, so avoid them immediately before reflexology. It's also not advisable to have a session after the client has eaten a heavy meal because reflexology affects circulation and may divert blood away from the digestive system where it is needed at this time.

When you are working on people who have never had reflexology before or know very little about it, show them a foot chart before you begin and briefly explain some of the principles. It makes the session less mysterious for them and later they can explain to others what they had done.

Always check the condition of the feet before you begin. Look for corns, cuts, bruises, and the like, and point these out before you begin so your partner doesn't think you caused them! Also, you'll want to work more gently on these areas or avoid them altogether.

It's more aesthetically pleasing to work on clean feet rather than dirty ones, so suggest to your partners (if they don't figure it out on their own) to wash their feet before a session. In the case of a spontaneous session, don't be embarrassed to just say frankly, "Go wash your feet first." You could also say, "I'll go wash my hands and you wash your feet." You could also tell them— and this is true—that washing the feet immediately before a session softens them and makes it easier for you to get into the points. Sometimes when Warren and I do reflexology on each other we soften the feet with hot wet towels. Wrapping each foot and letting the heat soak through can be a sensuous and loving act, and it allows each of us a moment to relax and talk over some of the things that have happened during the day.

Always wash your hands before and after reflexology. Clip and file your nails so that they won't snag or cut into the skin.

When you begin, note and adjust your posture so that your back is straight. Be aware of your posture as the session progresses. If you find yourself slumping or getting hunched over, straighten up. Breathe deeply as you work because you'll need plenty of oxygen for muscle performance and mental concentration. Besides, you don't want to end the session with tension in your own back or shoulders. Generally, I think you'll find that giving a reflexology session is relaxing for yourself as well as your partner. Steady, deep breathing, good posture, and centered, focused attention can give you a physical and spiritual boost.

Your attitude and intention before and during a session are extremely important because you are affecting your partner on many levels, not just the physical. Projecting confidence and strength, along with gentleness and sensitivity to the other, creates an emotional and spiritual bond between the two of you. As you do reflexology, you'll begin to realize how important this bonding is for healing to take place. It creates a oneness between the healer and receiver. The great value and beauty of hands-on therapies such as reflexology is that they provide what machines and sleek technology can never hope to achieve: the direct human contact, human warmth, and human love without which it is very difficult to be healthy and happy.

So clear your mind and center your attention before you begin. Breathe deeply, drawing in the healing energy of the universe. Make it your intention to be a channel of healing for the person you are working on, keeping in mind that it is not your own personal energy that passes into the feet you are holding. You are tapping into unlimited universal energy.

You may want to imagine the organs and glands you are working on the feet—see what they look like in the body and imagine them in perfect balance.

I find it helps to ground myself in love and concern for the client, and I visualize these positive emotions expressing themselves through my hands. Visualization such as this can help both client and reflexologist. Many healers and body workers attest to the importance of creative visualizations to keep themselves centered and focused while they apply their therapies. I know it works for me.

I heartily suggest that you share these warm, loving, positive thoughts and attitudes with your partner. You may find this extremely easy or extremely difficult to do. Some people can articulate spiritual and emotional sentiments to those they love; others find it hard to put such notions into words face to face with someone they know so well. They get embarrassed and feel ill at ease. It might help, therefore, to put what you want to say into the form of a moment's meditation that you both can share. It can be as simple as saying, "Let's be silent for a moment and concentrate on the healing that will take place and the energies that will pass through us," or something to that effect. It doesn't have to be syrupy or poetic. Just be honest about how you feel, and reflect for a moment on the health, love, and well-being you wish each other.

SESSION ORDER

My associates and I have developed a session order for a complete reflexology routine that we use with our clients. It is presented on the following pages, under two headings—Session Order: Relaxation Steps and Session Order: Reflexing Steps. Once you have learned each specific technique and you begin giving full sessions, you should stick to this order rather faithfully, but adjust it to fit the needs of individual partners, spending more time on trouble spots, coming back to reflex points that need special attention, and returning to relaxation techniques now and then, particularly after working a tender area.

SESSION PREPARATION

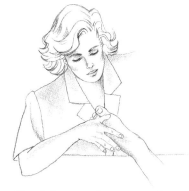

Center yourself, be clear on your intention. Become a channel for energy to flow through you. Breathe.

Check for cuts, bruises, and calluses.

SESSION ORDER: RELAXATION STEPS

Sitting

Greet both feet together:

top   bottom

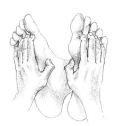

Stretch both legs together from hips

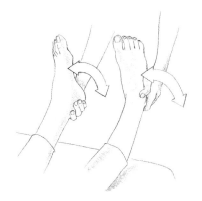

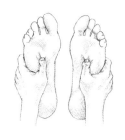

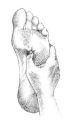

Thumb press on solar plexus—
both feet

Circular rotation on solar plexus

Hold solar plexus when
transferring feet

Ankle rocking (flipping) together

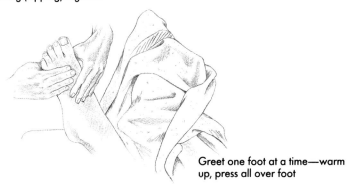

Greet one foot at a time—warm
up, press all over foot

Standing

Index finger slide on bottom of foot standing or
kneeling (if on floor) from shoulder line to up
around the heel (use body weight)

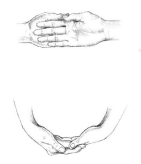

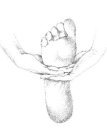

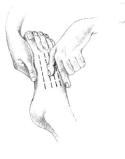

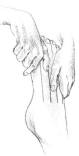

Troughing (thumb slides)

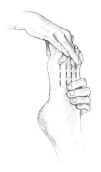 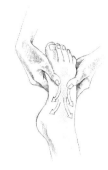 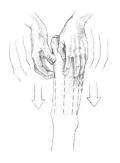 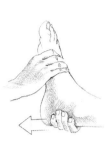

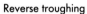

Reverse troughing

Alternating thumb rotations on top of the foot

Vibrating

Leg stretch out

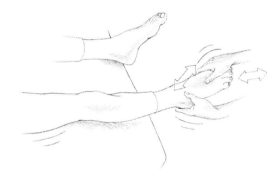 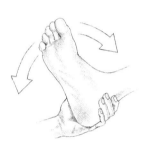

One-leg-stretch and bounce

Ankle rocking

Sitting

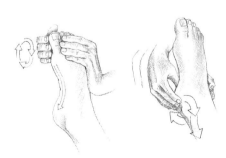 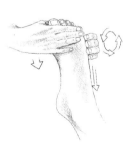 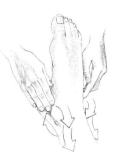

Fingertip rotations down inside of foot, up along Achilles tendon, and around anklebone

Fingertip rotations down the outside of foot, up along Achilles tendon, and around the anklebone

Circles around both anklebones together

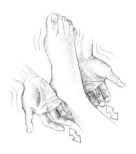

Ankle boogie

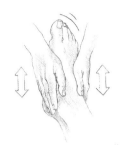

Palm rubdown and outsides
of thumbs on top of foot

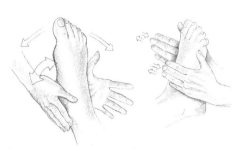

Foot boogie

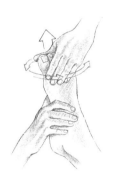

Toe rotations—all at once

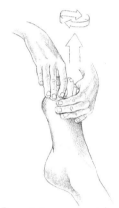

Toe rotations, separately—
traction, then rotate

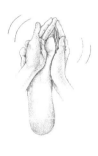

Toe boogie—use pinkies—then
stretch

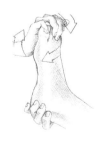

Ankle rotations—under

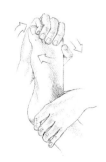

Ankle rotations—over

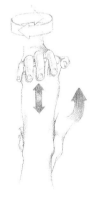

Achilles tendon stretch

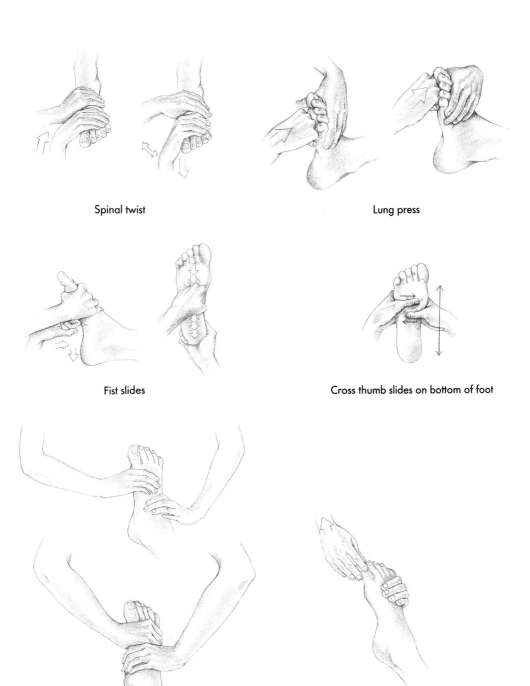

Spinal twist

Lung press

Fist slides

Cross thumb slides on bottom of foot

Wringing the foot

Toe stretches

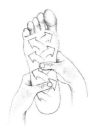

Alternating thumb rotations on bottom of foot

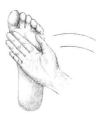

Slapping foot with back of hand

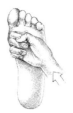

Punch with back of fist (no knuckles)

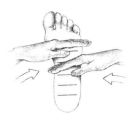

Karate chops

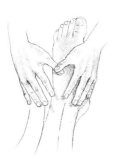

Breeze stroke

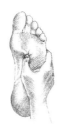

Thumb press on solar plexus—one foot

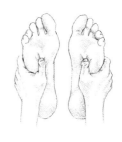

Thumb presses on solar plexus—both feet

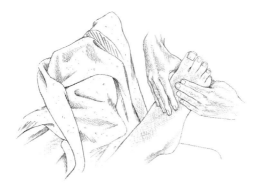

Release right thumb—cover foot and begin repeating relaxation on other foot. Cover foot. After completing foot relaxation, begin the reflexology session order.

SESSION ORDER: REFLEXING STEPS

WORK THE POINTS SUGGESTED BELOW ON ONE ENTIRE FOOT, THEN SWITCH AND WORK THE POINTS ON THE OTHER FOOT.

Begin with Left Foot

The illustrations below are demonstrated on the left foot. These techniques are also done on the right foot.

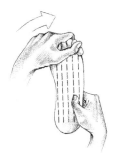

Thumb walk zones 5 through 1

CHEST/LUNG, HEART, SHOULDER, ARM

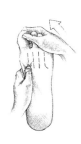

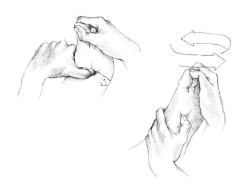

Thumb walk chest and lung area from diaphragm line to neck/ shoulder line

Thumb walk and rotate onto diaphragm line—both directions

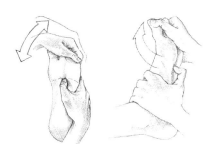

Flex and pivot onto diaphragm

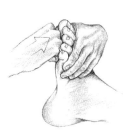
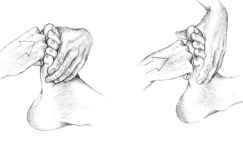

Lung press

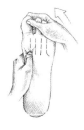

Thumb walk heart

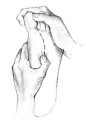

Thumb walk bronchial tube helper
to thyroid and esophagus

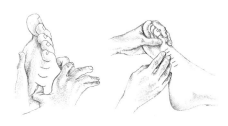

Thumb and finger walk shoulder
and arm

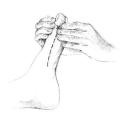

Finger walk thymus and thoracic
area of spine up to seventh
cervical

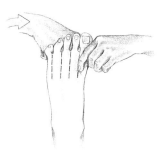

Finger walk front of foot—chest,
lymph drainage, inner ear, vocal
cords, mammary glands, and
shoulder blades—upper back

NECK, THYROID, THROAT

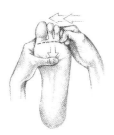 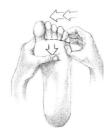 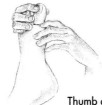

Thumb and finger walk neck/
shoulder line, going around to
front of foot—around front base
of big and little toes (in the joints)

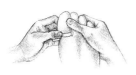

Thumb walk thyroid and
parathyroids

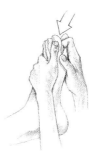

Hang on ridge of toes for
shoulder and neck line

HEAD

Thumb walk down
the five zones
of the big toe

Thumb walk down the smaller
toes, making three passes
on each

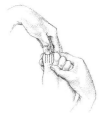 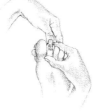 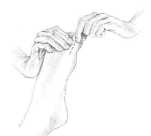

Thumb walk up bottom
of toes— sinus, eyes,
ears

Finger walk down front of
toes

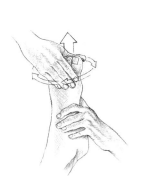

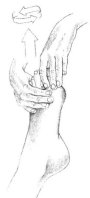

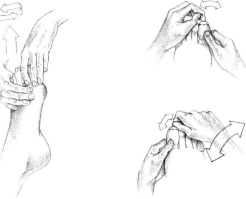

Stretch and rotate all toes together

Individually stretch and rotate toes

Finger roll and thumb roll brain

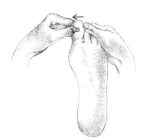

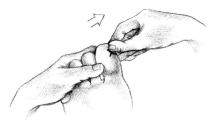

Hook and back-up on pituitary

Hook, and back-up on pineal/ hypothalamus

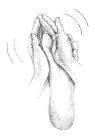

Toe boogie

PELVIC AREA TO WAIST—LEFT FOOT

Warm up heel—thumb walk in three directions

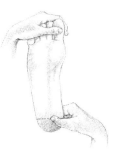

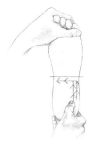

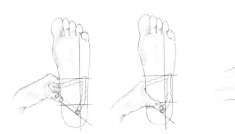

Thumb walk up descending colon

Thumb walk and rotate onto splenic flexure

Thumb walk across transverse colon

Thumb walk down and hook and back-up sigmoid flexure—left foot

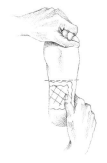

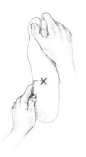

Thumb walk and pivot away small intestines on a diagonal, up and across—crosshatch in both directions from pelvic line to waist

Thumb walk bladder up ureters to kidney

WAIST TO DIAPHRAGM—LEFT FOOT ONLY

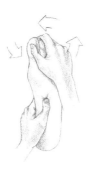

Rotate and pivot away onto kidney

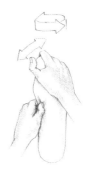

Rotate and pivot away onto adrenals

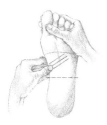

Thumb walk and pivot away on a diagonal (cross hatching) area from waist line to diaphragm covering liver, pancreas, and duodenum

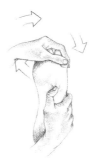

Rotate and pivot away onto spleen

PELVIC AREA TO WAIST

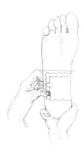

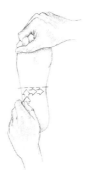

Hook and back-up ileocecal valve
and appendix

Thumb walk up ascending colon

Thumb walk across transverse
colon

Thumb walk and rotate onto
hepatic flexure

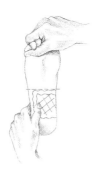

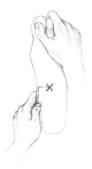

Thumb walk and pivot away on
small intestines on a diagonal, up
and across—crosshatch in both
directions from pelvic line to waist
line

Thumb walk bladder up ureters to
kidney

WAIST TO DIAPHRAGM • RIGHT FOOT ONLY

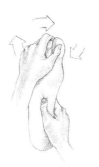

Rotate and pivot onto kidney

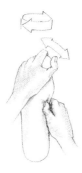

Rotate and pivot onto adrenals

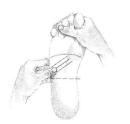

Thumb walk and pivot away on a
diagonal (crosshatching) area
from waist line to diaphragm
covering liver, pancreas, and
duodenum

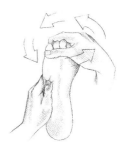

Rotate onto gallbladder

SPINE/BACK

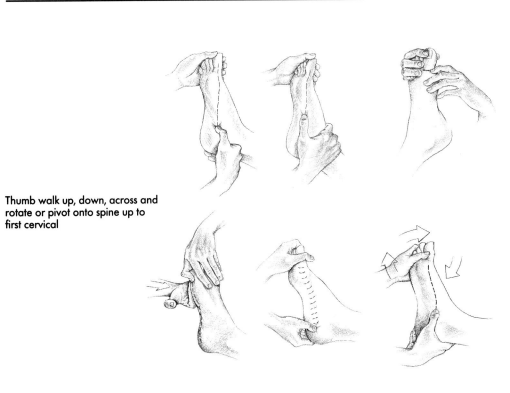

Thumb walk up, down, across and rotate or pivot onto spine up to first cervical

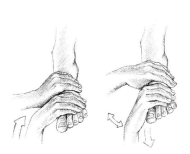

Spinal twist

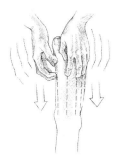

Vibrate down on front of foot

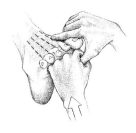

Finger walk down front of foot (mid-back)

LEG, KNEE, HIP, SCIATIC NERVE

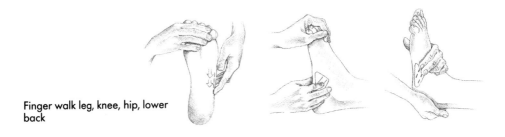

Finger walk leg, knee, hip, lower back

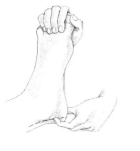

Finger walk up sciatic nerve—inside of ankle and leg (Achilles tendon area)

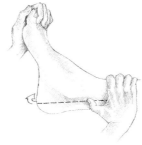

Thumb walk down sciatic nerve—inside of leg six inches above ankle

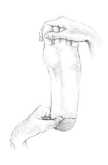

Thumb walk sciatic nerve across bottom of foot—work heel in all directions

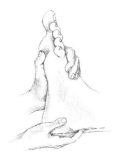

Finger walk up sciatic nerve—outside of ankle and leg (Achilles tendon area)

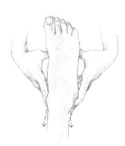

Work chronic area—sciatic, rectum, reproductive

REPRODUCTIVE

Rotate ankle:

—Under

—Over

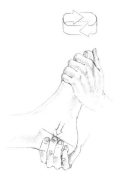

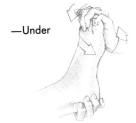

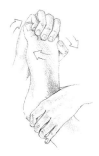

Rotate onto uterus, prostate; finger walk area

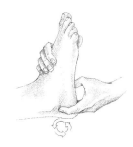

Small circular rotation movement onto ovaries, testicles

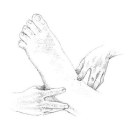

Finger walk lymph/groin, fallopian tubes, seminal vesicles

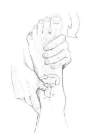

Rotate thumb into hollow at lymph/groin area

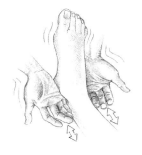

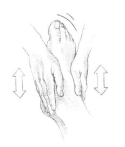

Ankle boogie, palm boogie

MORE RELAXATION TECHNIQUES

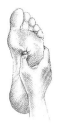

Solar plexus

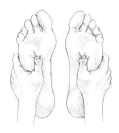

Thumb press solar plexus

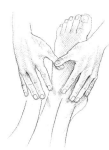

Breeze stroke

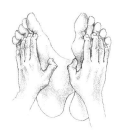

End with breeze strokes each foot
Relax both feet together

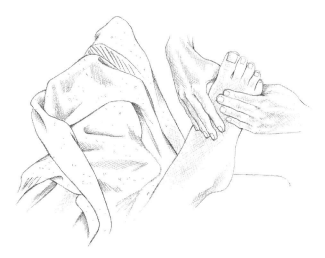

Repeat sequence to other foot

SESSION ORDER: SUMMARY

For easy reference, this section lists the steps that were illustrated on the previous pages.

Remember: Create a comfortable, relaxed environment and mood. Before the routine, prepare the materials needed such as washcloths, towels, cream, pillows, and a cover. Check your nail length. Work on children, the elderly, or the very ill with lighter pressure, for shorter lengths of time, and with more frequent sessions. Consistent sessions will create cumulative results.

Relaxation Steps

Center yourself, be clear on your intention.

Become a channel for energy to flow through you.

Breathe.

Check for cuts, bruises, calluses.

Begin relaxation techniques using a nongreasy cream. Start relaxation techniques on both feet. Then relax the entire left foot, and then the right.

Sitting

- Greet both feet together
    - -top
    - -bottom
- Stretch both legs together from hips
- Ankle rocking (flipping) together
- Thumb press on solar plexus

- Circular rotation on solar plexus
- Thumb press solar plexus when transferring feet
- Greet one foot at a time—warm up, press foot all over

Standing

- Index finger slide on bottom of foot standing or kneeling (if on floor) from shoulder line to heel and up behind heel (use body weight)
- Troughing (thumb slides)
- Reverse troughing

- Alternating thumb rotations on top of the foot—clockwise, counterclockwise
- Vibrating
- One leg stretch
- One leg bounce
- Ankle Rocking

Sitting

- Fingertip rotations down inside of foot, up along Achilles tendon, and around anklebone
- Fingertip rotations down the outside of foot, up along Achilles tendon, and around anklebone
- Circles around both anklebones together
- Ankle boogie

- Palm rub down and outsides of thumbs on top of foot
- Foot boogie
- Toe rotations—all at once
- Toe rotations, separately—traction then rotate
- Toe boogie—use pinkies—then stretch
- Under—ankle rotations

(Sitting cont.)

- Over—ankle rotations
- Achilles tendon stretch
- Spinal twist
- Lung press
- Fist slides
- Cross thumb slides on bottom of foot
- Wringing the foot
- Toe stretches
- Alternating thumb rotations on bottom of foot
- Slapping foot with back of hand
- Punch with back of fist (no knuckles)
- Karate chops
- Breeze stroke
- Thumb press on solar plexus—one foot
- Thumb presses on solar plexus—both feet
- Release right thumb—cover foot and begin repeating relaxation on the other foot. Cover foot. After completing foot relaxation, begin session order.

Reflexing Steps

Powder to absorb excess cream or perspiration.
Work the points suggested below on the entire left foot, then switch and work the points on the right foot.

BOTH FEET (One Foot at a Time)

- Thumb walk zones 5–1

CHEST/LUNG, HEART, SHOULDER, ARM

- Thumb walk chest and lung area from diaphragm line to neck/shoulder line
- Thumb walk and rotate onto diaphragm line—both directions
- Flex and pivot onto diaphragm
- Lung press
- Thumb walk bronchial tube and thyroid helper
- Thumb walk heart
- Thumb walk esophagus (left foot only)
- Thumb walk shoulder and arm
- Finger walk thymus and thoracic area of spine up to seventh cervical
- Finger walk front of foot—chest, lymph drainage, and mammary glands
- Shoulder blades—upper back

NECK, THYROID

- Hang on ridge of toes for shoulder and neckline
- Thumb and finger walk neck/shoulder line going around to front of foot—
- around front base of big and little toes (in the joints)
- Thumb walk thyroid and parathyroid

HEAD

- Thumb walk down back of toes— sinus, eyes, ears
- Thumb walk up back toes—sinus, eyes, ears
- Finger walk front of toes
- Stretch and rotate all toes together
- Individually stretch and rotate toes
- Finger roll and thumb roll brain
- Hook and back up on pituitary/ hypothalamus
- Hook and back up on pineal
- Toe boogie

From the pelvic area to the waist, and from the waist to the diaphragm, there are differences in the reflex areas and points of the left and right foot. These areas correspond to the locations of the various organs and glands in the body. Continue on left foot. (Skip this section when working on right foot.)

Points on Left Foot

PELVIC AREA TO WAIST

- Warm up heel—thumb walk in 3 directions
- Thumb walk down and hook and back up sigmoid colon—left foot
- Thumb walk up descending colon
- Thumb walk splenic flexure
- Thumb walk across transverse colon
- Thumb walk and pivot away small intestines on a diagonal, up and across—crosshatch in both directions from pelvic line to waist
- Thumb walk bladder up ureters to kidney

WAIST TO DIAPHRAGM

- Rotate and pivot away onto kidney
- Rotate and pivot away onto adrenals
- Thumb walk and pivot away on a diagonal—crosshatching area from waistline to diaphragm line, covering stomach and pancreas and duodenum
- Rotate and pivot away onto spleen
- Continue on left foot. Skip this section (points on right foot) until working pelvic area to waist on the right foot.

Points on Right Foot

PELVIC AREA TO WAIST

- Hook and back up appendix and ileocecal valve
- Thumb walk up ascending colon
- Thumb walk and rotate hepatic flexure
- Thumb walk across transverse colon
- Thumb walk and pivot away on small intestine on a diagonal, up and across
- Crosshatch in both directions from pelvic line to waist line
- Thumb walk bladder up ureters to kidney

WAIST TO DIAPHRAGM

- Rotate and pivot onto kidney
- Rotate and pivot onto adrenals
- Thumb walk and pivot away on a diagonal, crosshatching area from

  waist to diaphragm, covering liver, pancreas, and duodenum
- Rotate onto gallbladder

Both Feet (One at a Time)

SPINE/BACK

- Thumb walk up, down, across and rotate or pivot onto spine up to C1
- Spinal twist
- Vibrate down on front of foot
- Finger walk down front of foot (mid-back)

LEG, KNEE

- Thumb walk up and finger walk down outside of foot
- Finger walk leg, knee, and hip sciatic nerve helper
- Finger walk up inside of leg for sciatic nerve—six inches above ankle
- Thumb walk down sciatic nerve— inside of leg six inches above ankle
- Thumb walk sciatic nerve—bottom of foot
- Finger walk sciatic nerve and hip— outside of foot
- Work chronic area—sciatic, rectum, reproductive

REPRODUCTIVE

- Rotate ankle
    -under
    -over
- Rotate onto uterus, prostate, finger walk area
- Small circular rotation movement onto ovaries, testes, finger walk area
- Ankle boogie, palm boogie
- Finger walk lymph groin, fallopian tubes, seminal vesicles
- Rotate thumb into hollows at lymph groin area
- More relaxation techniques
- Repeat sequence to right foot
- Thumb press solar plexus
- Breeze stroke
- End by relaxing both feet together
- Solar plexus
- Breeze stroke

An Overview of an Alternate Session Order

- Relaxation techniques on both feet, then left foot, then right
- Thumb press solar plexus when transferring feet
- Thumb walk zones—left foot and then right foot—before working reflex areas
- Work reflex areas and points on entire left foot, then right, in the following order:
- Chest region
- Neck area
- Head region
- Spine, back area
- Knee, leg, hip, sciatic nerve areas, lower back
- Chronic area—sciatic nerve, rectum, and reproductive
- Reproductive points
- Internal organs and glands from pelvic area to waist
- Internal organs and glands from waist to diaphragm
- Integrate relaxation techniques through out session to relieve tender areas.
- Repeat routine on right foot. End with both feet.
- Solar plexus and breeze strokes

Now that you know how to go about giving a reflexology session, let's take a look at the many situations in daily life where reflexology can make a real difference in your health and well-being and that of your family and friends.

In the following chapters you will find routines we call "Good Steps" for specific ailments and conditions, as well as general advice for different categories of people. As you apply reflexology, you'll learn when and how often to give sessions, partially based on the receiver's need for them. Generally speaking, do the routines as needed, or at least once or twice a week. If you decide to give sessions daily or every other day, reduce the length of the session to approximately ten to twenty minutes (instead of a full session which usually runs thirty to sixty minutes). Some Good Steps routines will advise you specifically on frequency and duration.

CHAPTER FOUR

THE NATURE OF STRESS

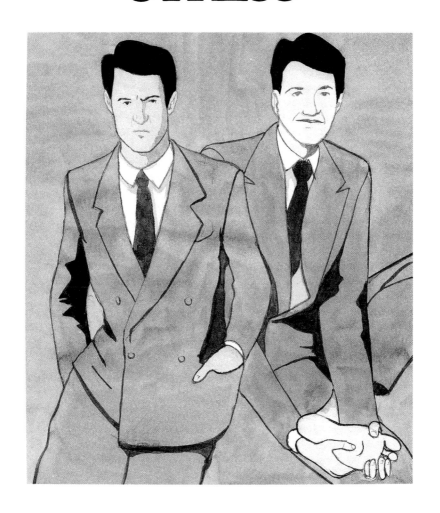

Two thousand years ago Plato pointed out that "the part can never be well unless the whole is well," and Western health care practitioners have been rediscovering that fact ever since. We do not live in a vacuum. Everything we do is interconnected to all the parts of our lives. Sickness and disease are not isolated phenomena existing in their own little corners of our world any more than are health and healing. Our state of health colors our entire life and is in turn influenced by all our activities, work and play, every relationship, the food we eat, our emotions and personalities, our physical living conditions. When you have a headache, you take it with you everywhere. It becomes part of your whole life. If part of you is ailing, all of you suffers. When you feel wonderful, that exuberance and joy permeates your relationships at work and play. Health is a tapestry through which all the threads of your life are intimately woven. You cannot pull one loose without unraveling or weakening the whole.

My personal belief is that reflexology can be a faithful source of strength and well-being, and should not be treated like a bottle of aspirin, sitting on a medicine shelf waiting for a headache to come along before you use it. It is more than just a remedy for unexpected ailments and sudden emergencies. In addition to being used when you aren't feeling well, reflexology is a method for enhancing your ordinary life by keeping you at the peak of your energies and creativity. It is a preventive measure to maintain a well-balanced body that can ward off illness and fatigue and maintain an optimal state of health and well-being so that whatever you do, you do with more enthusiasm, joy, and energy.

One of the key elements of life is stress. Because we are not living in a vacuum, we cannot avoid it. It is everywhere, but not as many people believe. Stress is not "out there" waiting to spring on us and disrupt our lives. The causes of stress are external, but stress itself is not in them, it is in us. Stress is the internal response we make to external changes and difficulties, whether real or imagined. The outside stressor or stimulus might be a boss reminding us of a deadline or just our imagination running wild, thinking about all the possible disasters of an upcoming dinner with in-laws. We experience stress when we lose faith in our ability to handle difficult situations, whether with the world in general or with specific people. At some point in a busy day this feeling of helplessness can strike any of us and we feel "stressed out."

The stress response is a signal that our body and all its major systems have been activated either to fight off the threatening condition or to flee from it.

This classic fight-flight reaction is not just in our heads. It reverberates throughout our entire body. Adrenaline is released, the heart rate quickens, breathing becomes shallower, blood vessels on the skin surface contract, blood pressure rises, digestion and intestinal processes shut down, muscles tense up, the stomach tightens. If all of these responses were under our conscious control, I would suggest that you try turning them all on right now and see how you feel. But of course you can't. For the most part, they are not under our direct control.

Nevertheless, you know what I'm talking about because you've felt them turn on automatically when you feel threatened by a stressful situation. Imagine the state of tension this mobilization plan can create throughout your body. None of these conditions are meant to persist for very long. The body couldn't stand it. They are short-term responses for short-term dangers. Unfortunately, we live in a society that is constantly confronting us with stressful situations. Some are very specific, such as traffic jams, and some are rather vague, generalized feelings of being at the mercy of other individuals and forces beyond our control, such as the perplexing state of the economy or the high level of violence in our society and the world at large. We feel helpless and victimized. Our stress response stays permanently turned on, even at low levels. We are on alert to resist. Such extreme mobilization can only be maintained so long without the body suffering from extreme exhaustion.

When the body prepares for fight or flight, it does so with a short-term goal in mind. The adrenal glands release adrenaline and noradrenaline into the bloodstream, two hormones which mimic the actions of nervous stimulation in a number of organs in the body. The heart rate increases, the blood vessels dilate in some areas and constrict in others, the rate of respiration increases, most digestive activities slow or stop altogether. We are prepared for a short burst of heightened activity.

In our modern-day lives, many stressors can trigger this fight-or-flight response, and most of them cannot be appropriately responded to with a short burst of activity. Over a period of time, adrenal stimulation with no discharge of energy will deplete essential vitamins and minerals from the system—substances especially important to the functioning of the immune system like vitamins B and C. Long-term adrenal activity can also affect blood pressure and cause a buildup of fatty substance of blood vessel walls, as well as damage the functioning of the digestive system.

The antidote to the state of alert generated by the stress response is relaxation, and reflexology is the key to relaxation. A relaxed and balanced body can heal itself. The *vis mediatrix naturae*—the healing power of nature—operates at its best when the body lets it operate. It requires rest, relaxation, and the gentle and natural flow of energy. A completely relaxed body cannot experience a negative emotion. We cannot feel anxiety, panic, hatred, fear, or bitterness when the body and its muscles are relaxed. Try it. When you are relaxed in a reflexology session, just try to *feel* bitterness or resentment toward someone. Of course the *idea* of bitterness or resentment can still cross your mind, but the emotional, feeling component is simply not there. Your body won't experience the negative emotion, nor will it jangle the nervous system, rev up the stress response, or wear down the immune system. The same is true of anxiety or fear. Your body and emotions cannot gear up for danger; you cannot resort to fight or flight when your body is relaxed. The remarkable thing about relaxation through reflexology is that you do not feel helpless as you relax. Quite the contrary: Reflexology instills confidence and the knowledge that you can cope with stress and stressful situations. You can *do* something to relieve the tensions of modern life. You have hope.

We all stand to benefit from giving relaxation a greater role in our lives. Unfortunately, we cannot just tell our bodies to relax. Giving orders does not guarantee that the body will obey; and if it doesn't, you will only generate more worry and reinforce your sense of helplessness. Persistent anxiety is harmful to the physical body, and it saps your overall ability to cope with frustration or engage in successful relationships with the people in your life.

Reflexology, however, is a guaranteed method of relaxing the body, composing the mind, and reenergizing and balancing the biological systems on which health depends. Reflexology can become the powerful antidote to stress, neutralizing and even preventing the insidious effects of stress: the headaches, high blood pressure, colds, eyestrain, indigestion, backaches, and other minor ailments that plague us.

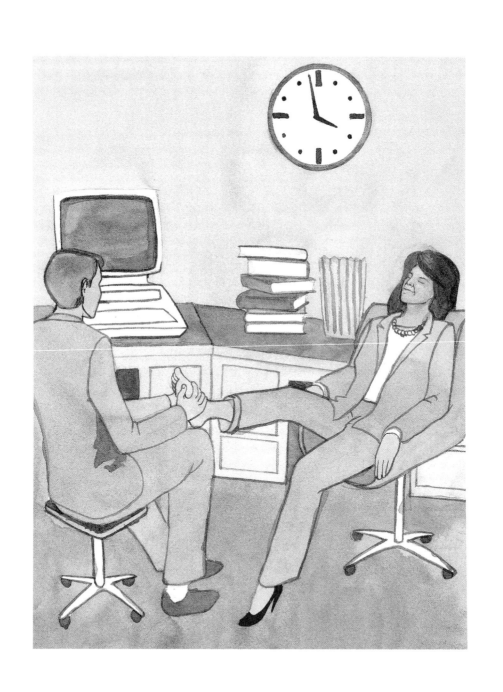

CHAPTER FIVE

GETTING AHEAD:

REFLEXOLOGY AT WORK AND SCHOOL

Career and job opportunities are constantly changing, along with the education and training required for them. As modern men and women we have to be on our toes to keep up with this ever-shifting milieu. Some of us worry that we have embarked upon lines of work or study that do not have the prestige or salaries that others expect of us. Others carve out career niches that become obsolete or are replaced by technology. Many corporate careerists step on a treadmill that keeps them constantly under pressure to advance up the corporate ladder or be eliminated. Women in business find that competing in a predominantly masculine world requires a stamina and determination not expected of their male counterparts; and men discover that to be the traditional "provider" for their families is harder to do with incomes that don't keep pace with skyrocketing prices. And throughout all the avenues of stress and tension, many of us suspect that ultimately career and salary are not the most important things about life. We find ourselves spending increasing amounts of time at tasks that don't satisfy us or allow us enough time to spend with family and friends.

Reflexology can ease these tensions and worries. While it will not take away the stimuli at work or school that cause stress, it will give you an outlet for shaking the deleterious effects of stress on the body and the immune system.

Reflexology helps people become less irritable and easier to work with. Others' quirky habits that normally drive you nuts become less annoying. You develop a more live-and-let-live attitude, so that even a jangling phone or the impatience of a coworker doesn't seem to matter so much. In a word, you become more tolerant.

HAPPY HOUR FOR THE FEET

Instead of the usual happy hour at the end of the day, a relaxing session of reflexology at home with a loved one can achieve the same effect—even better—without the danger of your becoming hooked on alcohol or drugs.

Ann, one of my students and a nurse, had a boyfriend who worked for a motion picture company and often came home tired and frustrated. The first thing he wanted to do was "pop a beer." Ann knew that he was putting on weight because of his evening happy hours. The two of them enjoyed this time together very much, but at the same time, she knew that his nightly beers weren't doing him any good. After a few reflexology classes, she felt confident enough to grab his feet first, before he could grab a beer. And thus a new tradition was born for them! Now they do reflexology on each other every night before dinner, instead of unwinding with a drink.

Remember: Before each routine in this chapter, set up the environment as described in Chapter Three. Prepare the materials needed such as lotion, towel, and cornstarch. Create the appropriate mood with lighting and music. Review the person's health history. Check the feet for cuts, bruises, sores, corns, or calluses. If necessary, clean the feet with a warm washcloth or handiwipe. Clear and center yourself.

GOOD STEPS: FOR OVERCOMING FATIGUE

Each session should last 20 minutes and be done whenever you feel tired. For overall energy, schedule sessions at least twice a week.

1. Relax both feet with relaxation techniques, and end by a thumb press on the solar plexus point in both feet. Relax each foot separately.

2. Thumb walk up the five zones of one foot and work the points suggested below.

3. Thumb walk up the five zones of the other foot and work the points suggested below.

4. Integrate relaxation techniques throughout the session as needed to help your partner relax when you encounter tender spots.

REFLEX AREA	TECHNIQUE	RATIONALE
DIAPHRAGM	Rotate onto thumb	• Promote deeper breathing, which increases oxygen intake and relaxes central nervous system
HEART	Thumb walk	• Promote steady heart rate and better circulation
THYROID AND HELPER AREA TO THYROID	Thumb walk and finger walk	• Balance metabolic rate
BRAIN	Finger roll	• Regulate all physical processes, including sleep and wakefulness • Balance central nervous system which can get overstimulated when fatigued
PITUITARY	Hook & back up	• Assist balancing endocrine functions
SPINE	Thumb walk up, down & across	• Regulate nerve impulses • Relieve muscle tension
PANCREAS	Thumb walk	• Increase energy through balancing blood sugar levels
SPLEEN, LYMPH/ GROIN	Rotate onto thumb	• Facilitate delivery of nutrients to and removal of wastes from body tissues
LIVER	Thumb walk and pivot on diagonal	• Release energy in the form of glucose into the bloodstream • Formulate blood constituents
ADRENALS	Rotate onto thumb	• Stimulate gland for release of energy-related hormones
ENTIRE FOOT	Karate chops, punch and slap	• Stimulate, wake up, and enliven the entire body

• Do relaxation techniques and thumb press on the solar plexus point in both feet, and end with breeze strokes.

Suggested Visualization:

Let your partner see herself taking an "energy shower" under a secluded, crystal-clear blue waterfall. If your partner likes, play Vivaldi's *The Four Seasons*, Bach's *Brandenburg Concertos*, or the gently invigorating music of her choice during the session.

SEDENTARY ACHES AND PAINS

Many sedentary jobs are deceiving. On the surface they look calm and quiet, but they generate seething cauldrons of internal turmoil and anxiety. Office workers, executives, and students spend long, fatiguing hours sitting at desks or tables—an "activity" which can sap energy as ruthlessly as farmwork or household chores. In fact, sedentary jobs are even more insidious precisely because they produce stress without the physical activity to release it. It is interesting that people who sit for long hours frequently complain of undifferentiated stress—stress that has no apparent cause or solution. It sneaks up on us in the midst of our normal business day, tightening our necks and shoulders, producing headaches and upset stomachs, leaving us feeling helpless and tense. Not even stress researchers understand this kind of stress completely.

Different people experience stress in different parts of the body. Wherever it catches you, locate the section and zone in your foot that correspond to that area, and work them thoroughly.

GOOD STEPS: FOR EYE, NECK, AND SHOULDER STRAIN

Each session should last 20 to 30 minutes and be done whenever you feel tension from sitting too long.

1. Relax both feet with relaxation techniques, and end by a thumb press on the solar plexus point in both feet. Relax each foot separately.

2. Thumb walk up the five zones of one foot and work the points suggested below.

3. Thumb walk up the five zones of the other foot and work the points suggested below.

4. Integrate relaxation techniques throughout the session as needed to help your partner relax when you encounter tender spots.

REFLEX AREA	TECHNIQUE	RATIONALE
LUNGS AND CHEST	Lung press	• Deepen and improve breathing
SHOULDER	Thumb walk	• Relax shoulder muscles
NECK	Thumb walk, finger walk, and hang on ridge	• Relax neck and cervicals in the spine
NECK	Toe rotation	• Relax and loosen neck
NECK AND HEAD	Toe boogie	• Relax and loosen neck and head muscles
SINUS AND EYE AREAS	Finger walk	• Relax optic nerve • Alleviate sinus congestion
PITUITARY	Hook & back-up	• Stimulate all glands to help them to function at a more optimal level
SPINE (especially cervical spine and between toes)	Thumb walk up, down, & across	• Improve all nerve responses
SPINE	Spinal twist	• Stretch spine
KIDNEYS	Rotate onto thumb	• Stimulate zones 2 and 3, which are the same zones as the eyes
ADRENALS	Rotate onto thumb	• Balance adrenaline levels in the muscles • Reduce muscle fatigue
ENTIRE FOOT	Foot boogie	• Relax entire foot and body

• Do relaxation techniques and thumb press on the solar plexus point in both feet, and end with breeze strokes.

Suggested Visualization:

Let your partner imagine a private, icy blue "healing tent" lowering over his head and shoulders. Have him imagine this cooling, refreshing environment gently polishing all the tension away. Try listening to piano music by Debussy during the session, too.

ENERGY REFUELING

Business people have adopted some of the quick remedies that students have practiced for years, such as knocking off a couple hours in the afternoon to jog or play a game of racketball. But not everyone has those opportunities. All you may have time for is a ten-minute break or a half-hour lunch. In this case, reflexology is the answer. It will relieve the blockages of circulation and energy that occur when you work with shoulders curled over your chest and your head dropped. Remember that breathing becomes shallow in this position, so when you pause for a reflexology break, sit back, let your chest expand, and breathe deeply.

One of the great benefits for office workers, students, and executives is the new type of energy that comes immediately after a satisfying reflexology session. My clients tell me they always return to their jobs with a different quality of energy to replace the nervous, fidgety energy that characterizes so much indoor activity. They claim they are more creative. They accomplish more, their productivity increases, and they are able to concentrate better on their tests or at "boring" meetings.

GOOD STEPS: FOR BUILDING UP ENERGY RESERVES

Each session should last 30 to 50 minutes and be done daily. After you notice improvement, reduce sessions to twice a week.

1.   Relax both feet with relaxation techniques, and end by a thumb press on the solar plexus point in both feet. Relax each foot separately.

2.   Thumb walk up the five zones of one foot and work the points suggested below more vigorously than usual.

3.   Thumb walk up the five zones of the other foot and work the points suggested below more vigorously than usual.

4.   Integrate relaxation techniques throughout the session as needed to help your partner relax when you encounter tender spots.

REFLEX AREA	TECHNIQUE	RATIONALE
DIAPHRAGM	Thumb walk and rotate onto thumb	• Send oxygen to cells • Open breathing • Free energy blocks
NECK/SHOULDER LINE	Thumb walk	• Relax neck muscles • Increase energy and blood supply
NECK AND HEAD	Toe boogie	• Relax and loosen neck and head muscles
THYROID AND PARATHYROID	Thumb walk across	• Balance metabolic rate • Regulate calcium in blood to improve nerve function
HELPER AREA TO THE THYROID	Thumb walk up and across	• Help the thyroid function better
NECK	Toe rotation	• Relax and loosen neck muscles
CERVICAL AREA AROUND TO FRONT OF TOE	Finger walk	• Relax the shoulder muscles • Reduce tension
BRAIN	Roll and rock	• Stimulate blood supply to the brain • Regulate nerve activity
PITUITARY	Hook & back-up	• Stimulate other endocrine glands to function more effectively
PANCREAS	Thumb walk across	• Regulate blood sugar
LIVER	Thumb walk on a diagonal	• Detoxify blood • Formation of blood constituents
KIDNEYS	Rotate onto thumb	• Filter waste products and control blood pressure • In Chinese medicine, kidneys are the seat of energy reserves
ADRENALS	Thumb walk, rotate onto thumb, and pivot	• Stimulate production of epinephrine for energy pick-up

• Do relaxation techniques and thumb press on the solar plexus point in both feet, and end with breeze strokes.

Suggested Visualization:

Have your partner imagine her energy as a glorious, fragrant pile of red, orange, and yellow autumn leaves resting at the bottom of the backbone. As the session progresses, have your partner imagine the wind is whirling those leaves of energy into a cyclone and up through her whole body, finally dissolving into her very being and infusing it with energy, joy, and confidence.

One of my clients liked reflexology so much that he organized a "foot break" at the large company he works for. He taught the basics to several people in his department, and now, instead of breaking for coffee in the afternoon when their energy levels are low, they meet in the lounge and take off their shoes to give each other reflexology. They all like the quick, relaxing pick-me-up. As an unexpected side benefit, the air in the lounge became fresher since none of them needs to smoke during the break. And what's more, the emotional atmosphere in the room has changed too. In the past, they used to gripe about the usual office problems. Now the lounge is quiet, almost meditative, and a lot more conducive to peace of mind.

VACATION STRESS

Some people find it difficult to relax and enjoy themselves, even on vacation or when they travel. The disruption of their usual routines can trigger the stress response, and they end up with headaches, upset stomachs, insomnia, or tight necks—even while supposedly relaxing by the poolside. Travel is quite stressful for many people. Jet lag, an unfamiliar environment, new customs to figure out, strange food, strange people, lack of exercise and dehydration from sitting in a car or plane too long, worry about what's going on at home or back in the office—all these can put pressure on the nervous system in subtle ways. So be alert to these stress-producing situations and make reflexology part of your travel plans.

Personally, I'm not a very enthusiastic traveler. In a car or plane, I can get queasy and bored after a short distance. But what I usually do is slip off my shoes and work on my feet a little to take my mind off the journey. Often, if the trip is long enough, I can fall asleep and that always helps pass the time.

GOOD STEPS: FOR TRAVEL STRESS

Each session should last 30 to 50 minutes and be done whenever possible before, during, and after traveling.

1. Relax both feet with relaxation techniques, and end by a thumb press on the solar plexus point in both feet. Relax each foot separately.

2. Thumb walk up the five zones of one foot and work the points suggested below.

3. Thumb walk up the five zones of the other foot and work the points suggested below.

4. Integrate relaxation techniques throughout the session as needed to help your partner relax when you encounter tender spots.

REFLEX AREA	TECHNIQUE	RATIONALE
LUNGS AND CHEST	Thumb walk vertically up zones	• Regulate breathing
LUNGS AND CHEST	Lung press	• Relax chest region and ease breathing
ARMS AND SHOULDERS	Thumb walk up	• Reduce muscle tension (especially if carrying luggage)
NECK	Thumb walk across	• Relax strained neck muscles
NECK AREA	Finger walk around	• Open up cervical vertebrae for better nerve flow
NECK	Toe rotation	• Relax and loosen neck muscles
NECK AND HEAD	Toe boogie	• Relax and loosen neck and head muscles

EYES AND EARS	Thumb walk down	• Reduce eyestrain • Strengthen equilibrium
BRAIN	Finger roll	• Clear the mind • Soothe nerve impulses
PITUITARY	Hook & back-up	• Stimulate glands so that they work more efficiently
SPINE	Thumb walk up, down, across	• Reinforce good posture • Balance nervous system
SPINE	Spinal twist	• Loosen and improve circulation to spine
HIP, KNEE, LEG, LOWER-BACK TRIANGLE	Finger walk	• Alleviate stress from sitting
SPLEEN	Rotate onto thumb	• Activate lymphatics • Spleen was considered by ancient civilizations to be the organ by which we acclimate to new environments
INTESTINES	Thumb walk in several directions on a diagonal	• Aid digestion and reduce possibility of constipation
ENTIRE FOOT	Cross thumb slide	• Soothe entire foot and body
ADRENALS	Rotate and pivot onto thumb	• Balance adrenaline release • Secrete hormones to regulate water, mineral balance, metabolism
ENTIRE FOOT	Karate chops, punch, and slap	• Stimulate, wake up, and enliven the body

- Do relaxation techniques and thumb press on the solar plexus point in both feet, and end with breeze strokes.

Suggested Visualization:

Let your partner imagine he is riding a beautiful green flying carpet, or on the back of a swan. Have your partner see the carpet or swan propelling him gently and effortlessly toward his destination.

REDUCING SICK DAYS

Many modern jobs are "head" jobs; that is, people no longer work with their bodies but with their minds. A steady routine of mental work at a desk day after day can take its toll on the immune system. Accountants, lawyers, secretaries, students, and other professionals, whether engaged in routine assignments or ones that are highly original and creative, need to get "out of their heads" now and then. Reflexology is a gentle way to do that, similar to the more strenuous techniques of physical exercise. It lets you indulge and get lost in the body for an hour or so, just as you do in sports. It improves circulation and can keep you healthy so that you miss fewer days of work.

GOOD STEPS: FOR BOOSTING THE IMMUNE SYSTEM

Each session should last 20 to 30 minutes and be scheduled 2 to 3 times per week.

1.   Relax both feet with relaxation techniques, and end by a thumb press on the solar plexus point in both feet. Relax each foot separately.

2.   Thumb walk up the five zones of one foot and work the points suggested below.

3.   Thumb walk up the five zones of the other foot and work the points suggested below.

4.   Integrate relaxation techniques throughout the session as needed to help your partner relax when you encounter tender spots.

REFLEX AREA	TECHNIQUE	RATIONALE
CHEST	Thumb walk	• Reduce nervous or rapid heartbeat
THYMUS	Thumb walk	• Stimulate immune activity, i.e., production of antibodies and blood cleansing

LYMPH DRAIN/NECK AREA	Finger walk	• Return lymph to general circulation
NECK	Hang on ridge	• Stimulate circulation to neck, throat, and thyroid, where there are a lot of lymph glands
THYROID AND TONSILS	Thumb walk	• Strengthen immune system structures
PITUITARY	Hook & back-up	• Stimulate all glands to rebalance hormone levels • Produce somatotropin, which stimulates production of lymphocytes
SPLEEN	Rotate onto thumb and thumb walk	• Activate immune structures which help fight infection
LIVER	Thumb walk across and diagonally	• Neutralize toxins in the blood
ADRENALS	Rotate onto thumb and thumb walk	• Stimulate energy • Combat inflammation
ILEOCECAL VALVE	Hook & back-up	• If it is open, this can cause toxicity and flu-like symptoms • Mucus control and release; part of cleansing process
INTESTINAL AREA	Thumb walk diagonally	• Help eliminate waste
KIDNEYS	Rotate and pivot onto thumb	• Reduce fluid retention • Stimulate waste elimination
LYMPH/GROIN AREA	Finger walk across, ankle rotations, rotate onto thumb	• Activate immune structures which help fight infection
ENTIRE FOOT	Cross thumb slide	• Soothe entire foot and body

•   Do relaxation techniques and thumb press on the solar plexus point in both feet, and end with breeze strokes.

Suggested Visualization:

Let your partner see and feel a bright pink light flowing through the body. Have her feel that light soothing and then energizing the immune system. If you like, also suggest to your partner that she imagine the sound of soft bells gently stimulating the immune system awake.

In subsequent sessions, have your partner see the immune cells attacking and destroying infection in whatever images are most powerful. Maybe the immune cells are beautiful tropical fish eating up green algae in a blue lagoon. Perhaps they're knights in shining armor. Encourage your partner to be playful, and to let her imagination flow.

TIME PRESSURE

One of the chief causes of stress is a sense of time pressure produced by the necessity of meeting deadlines. Trying to beat the clock always generates tension, but the situation becomes even more demoralizing when poor health, sleepiness, or lack of concentration makes jobs take longer than you had planned and you realize that you are getting even further behind. Face it, sedentary work is always "behind" work in more ways than one! Very few people seem to be right on schedule. By faithfully treating yourself to reflexology during the course of the week, you'll eliminate many of the conditions that accompany a stressful life and you'll not lose valuable time because of poor mental or physical health.

Some people, especially the classic "Type A" personalities, claim they thrive on deadlines and do their best work under pressure. I don't doubt that they do. The questions in my mind, however, are: Is that the only way they can perform best? Do they have to risk heart attacks and strokes just to be successful? What is more important—their work projects or their health? Type A people don't have to remain Type A. They can learn by imitating Type B behavior—slow down, take things more calmly and put less stress on their overworked nervous and immune systems. Believing that they will do well only under pressure is precisely that—a belief. And we are all capable of changing our beliefs and the behavior that arises from them. Reflexology can be a valuable tool in learning how to slow down and experience how good you can feel when relaxed, unhurried, at peace with your body and yourself.

GOOD STEPS: FOR CALMING YOURSELF DOWN

Each session should last at least 10 minutes and be done whenever you feel tense or anxious.

1. Relax both feet with relaxation techniques, and end by a thumb press on the solar plexus point in both feet. Relax each foot separately.

2. Thumb walk up the five zones of one foot and work the points suggested below.

3. Thumb walk up the five zones of the other foot and work the points suggested below.

4. Integrate relaxation techniques throughout the session as needed to help your partner relax when you encounter tender spots.

REFLEX AREA	TECHNIQUE	RATIONALE
CHEST/LUNG/HEART AREA	Thumb walk vertically up zones	• Regulate breathing and heart rate
DIAPHRAGM LINE	Thumb walk across and rotate onto thumb	• Aid in natural and easy breathing
LUNGS AND CHEST	Lung press	• Relax chest and deepen breathing
ENTIRE FOOT	Wringing	• Relax entire foot and body
NECK	Toe rotation	• Relax and loosen neck muscles
PITUITARY	Hook & back-up	• Balance all glandular functioning
NECK AND HEAD	Toe boogie	• Relax and loosen neck and head muscles
ADRENALS	Thumb walk and rotate onto thumb	• Balance energy levels • Open airways in lungs for better oxygen/carbon dioxide exchange
SPINE	Spinal twist	• Reduce stress on nervous system

• Do relaxation techniques and thumb press on the solar plexus point in both feet, and end with breeze strokes.

Suggested Visualization:

Let your partner imagine he is lying on a bed of soft, fragrant magnolia or rose petals. Then ask him to feel a pair of great, soft hands quietly smoothing his body and mind toward tranquility. If you like, play a recording of American spirituals by an artist like Miriam Makeba during the session.

GOOD STEPS: FOR HIGH OR LOW BLOOD PRESSURE

Each session should last 15 to 20 minutes and be scheduled 3 times a week.

1. Relax both feet with relaxation techniques, and end by a thumb press on the solar plexus point in both feet. Relax each foot separately.

2. Thumb walk up the five zones of one foot and work the points suggested below.

3. Thumb walk up the five zones of the other foot and work the points suggested below.

4. Integrate relaxation techniques throughout the session as needed to help your partner when you encounter tender spots.

REFLEX AREA	TECHNIQUE	RATIONALE
HEART AND ENTIRE CHEST REGION	Thumb walk all directions	• Regulate and strengthen cardiovascular functions
DIAPHRAGM	Thumb walk and rotate onto thumb	• Deepen breathing • Bring oxygen to cells
LUNGS AND CHEST	Lung press	• Relax chest region
THYROID AND PARATHYROID	Thumb walk	• Regulate metabolism and pulse rates • Balance calcium levels
PITUITARY	Hook & back-up	• Help regulate endocrine glandular processes
SPINE	Thumb walk up and down	• Balance nervous system
LIVER	Thumb walk	• Improve portal circulation
KIDNEYS	Rotate onto thumb	• Reduce water retention and process wastes out of the body
ADRENALS	Rotate and pivot onto thumb	• Control sodium and potassium levels that affect blood pressure

- Do relaxation techniques and thumb press on the solar plexus point in both feet, and end with breeze strokes.

Suggested Visualization:

For high blood pressure, let your partner imagine a shining golden liquid passing through her entire circulatory system, calming it and slowing it. Pay special attention to the golden liquid as it passes through the head and the heart, concentrating on it pooling in these areas and soothing them before it continues on its way.

For low blood pressure, let your partner imagine that a shining green liquid is filling her with energy and vigor. Pay special attention to the heart and the solar plexus areas as the liquid flows through the passageways there.

Whether at work, at school, or at home, busy people need to monitor their health, conserve energy for important occasions, and reduce stress as much as possible. With so many stimuli to produce stress and wear us out—and down—we owe it to ourselves and the people we live and work with to preserve our physical and emotional integrity and function at our very best. Reflexology can be the means of bringing balance and order into your life and supplying you with the energy and stamina needed to live life more fully.

CHAPTER SIX

SOLE MATES: COUPLES' REFLEXOLOGY

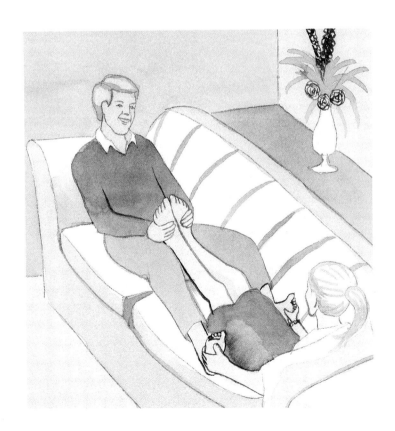

Believe it or not, many of my clients tell me that reflexology is "as good as sex." Some clients are a little more guarded and will only admit that it's "second to sex." And those who don't want to talk about sex may say that reflexology is "ecstasy" or "heaven." However they feel comfortable putting it, they're all onto something I always suspected: a reflexology high and a sexual high have a lot in common. Of course, I've always thought so, but then I'm prejudiced. Now, based on testimony from countless men and women, I firmly believe that there is a relationship between the two. Not only do people use the same language to describe similarities between reflexology and sex, but reflexology can be used to enhance sexual pleasure and sexual relationships. And couples who do reflexology in conjunction with making love say that they never realized "it" could be so good. "It" of course is not reflexology! (Although reflexology between lovers is also great!)

REFLEXOLOGY AND SEX

First, let me clear up a common misunderstanding about all this. Working the points on the feet for the sexual organs does not turn people on. In fact, because these points lie on the bony part of the foot below the ankle where the skin is thin, most people experience a little tenderness there. No, reflexology is not a long-lost sexual technique that the writers of the *Kamasutra* overlooked.

What happens is that reflexology relaxes you physically, clears your mind of worries, and reduces tension in all parts of the body so that you are more responsive and sensitive to sexual pleasure. Reflexology doesn't turn you on, but it gets you ready to be turned on by whatever turns you on! You can make love with greater freedom and spontaneity, with more energy and suppleness, giving yourself more wholly to the rituals of love that you and your partner enjoy.

Furthermore, reflexology is a great form of nonverbal communication, just like sex can be. Stimulating areas on the foot and creating pleasurable sensations on very deep levels is comparable to the physical stimulation and pleasure couples experience while making love. The "heaven" and "ecstasy" that people use to describe how they feel after sex—and reflexology—indicates the intense fulfillment we can feel after a great relaxing physical and emotional release.

Another similarity between making love and reflexology is the total immersion into the other person. Reflexology is done best when you can forget yourself and enter into the peace and relaxation you are giving your partner, such that you are truly giving of yourself. It moves your consciousness outside yourself, and allows you to tap into the higher sources of universal energy and love that you share with your partner. You see each other as totally complete and whole; you relate to each other in terms of your higher selves, even though, paradoxically, you are working with each other's physical self. But that's why it's such a total feeling of wholeness: you are loving each other on the physical and spiritual planes simultaneously. You are grounded and yet able to transcend the physical relationship you share with each other.

Couples who are just getting to know each other sexually, on an ongoing basis can use reflexology to overcome the nervousness and uncertainty that often characterizes new relationships. A couple's sexual harmony does not always develop overnight. If you have just moved in with your partner, you may discover all kinds of stress and tension that were not anticipated when you only saw each other a couple of times a week. Even seeing each other every day when you live apart is not the same as living and loving successfully under the same roof. It takes time and commitment.

You are sharing more than just geographical space. You share head and heart space as well, and that takes some getting used to. For young people living away from home for the first time as well as older persons set in their so-called ways, learning to live with another human being can also take practice. Reflexology is the perfect way to get over the stressful moments, loosen up, and learn to relax with each other. It's great foreplay and afterplay!

John, a former student of mine, moved in with his girlfriend while he was still in training to become a professional reflexologist. Neither of them had ever lived with anyone before and, consequently, they were both used to having their personal space and using it however they wished. Imagine the adjustment when they coupled up in a small studio apartment! They soon discovered that they both got home at about the same time each day so neither had a chance to unwind and be alone for a little while in the apartment before the other came in, something they both secretly longed for. So John suggested that the first thing they do when they got home each afternoon was a little reflexology on each other. His girlfriend was skeptical at first, but in no time they both found that a half hour of reflexology created a quiet "inner space" for themselves that

made up for their lack of personal "outer space." Soon they began looking forward to their late-afternoon reflexology sessions so much that it
became inconceivable to either one of them to want to be home alone
without the other. Today they both attribute reflexology to helping them
make this crucial adjustment in living together.

Remember: before each routine in this chapter, set up the environment as
described in Chapter Three. Prepare the materials needed, such as lotion,
towel, and cornstarch. Create the appropriate mood with lighting and music.
Review the person's health history. Check the feet for cuts, bruises, sores,
corns, or calluses. If necessary, clean the feet, with a warm washcloth or
handiwipe. Clear and center yourself.

GOOD STEPS: FOR LOVEMAKING

Each session should last 15 to 20 minutes, before, during, or after making
love. Use slow, sensual movements and a lot of relaxation techniques.

1. Relax both feet with relaxation techniques, and end by a thumb press on
    the solar plexus point in both feet. Relax each foot separately.

2. Thumb walk up the fives zones of one foot and work the points sug-
    gested below.

3. Thumb walk up the five zones of the other foot and work the points
    suggested below.

4. Integrate relaxation techniques throughout the session as needed to help
    your partner relax when you encounter tender spots.

REFLEX AREA	TECHNIQUE	RATIONALE
CHEST, LUNGS AND SHOULDER	Thumb walk	• Strengthen circulation to the heart • Open up breathing and relax shoulder muscles
LUNGS AND CHEST	Lung press	• Deepen breathing
NECK, THYROID	Thumb walk	• Relax neck muscles • Stimulate metabolism • Reduce muscle tension
NECK	Toe rotation	• Relax and loosen neck muscles
ENTIRE FOOT	Wringing	• Relax entire foot and body
BRAIN	Finger roll	• Regulate physical and mental reactions
PITUITARY	Hook & back-up	• Normalize glandular functions
ENTIRE FOOT	Thumb rotations	• Relax entire foot and body
ADRENALS	Rotate onto thumb	• Balance energy level
FALLOPIAN TUBES/ SEMINAL VESICLES	Ankle rotation	• Stimulate groin, fallopian tubes, and seminal vesicles
UTERUS/PROSTATE	Rotate onto finger	• Balance sex hormone production and release
OVARIES/TESTICLES	Small circular finger rotations	• Help produce hormones to improve vitality
ENTIRE FOOT	Vibrations	• Relax entire foot and body

• Do relaxation techniques and thumb press on the solar plexus point in both feet, and end with breeze strokes.

Suggested Visualization:

Have your partner imagine himself looking beautiful and desirable or feeling comfortable and safe as he lies in the center of a beautiful, rich, purple and red velvet carpet.

SEXUAL DYSFUNCTIONS

Serious problems can plague a relationship if one or both parties suffer from sexual dysfunction. Impotency and premature ejaculation in men and frigidity in women are common sexual problems, and in most cases, the source of the dysfunction is emotional or psychological. Sex therapists and physicians commonly point to stress as the major culprit. Of course, knowing that these problems are stress-related doesn't make them any easier to overcome. Worrying about the elusive nature of stress can simply escalate the tension. A vicious circle results that is often hard to break out of. Anything that will help the couple relax, lead a less stressful life, and ward off fatigue, or anything that will help them handle stress in a positive and healthy way may be the solution. Reflexology can do just that, and it's a lot safer than resorting to drugs or extended happy hours in the evening.

Al, a sixty-seven-year-old student of mine, was a cheerful and optimistic man who on the first day of class shared a personal secret with everyone in class. He had been impotent for three years. A warm, loving person, he was nevertheless somewhat tense and worried about this, in addition to problems he was having with his heart, for which he was on medication. After learning the basics, Al began doing reflexology on many of his friends in the retirement community where he and his wife lived. This made an incredible improvement in his life. He got valuable reinforcement and praise from his reflexology work among older people and he enjoyed associating with younger people once a week in class. After two months of weekly classes, getting his own feet worked on, and the new self-confidence he acquired by doing reflexology on others, he came into class one day with a sly-fox grin on his face, and announced that he had noticed what he proudly called "significant changes" in his sexual life!

A former client of mine confided in me once that she thought she was sexually dysfunctional. The way she put it was that once she and her husband got going, everything was great, but she suffered tremendous anxiety before they actually started to make love. She figured part of her problem was that she was an extremely busy woman, on the go all day, hardly ever stopping to catch her breath. In fact, from the way she described herself, she was a workaholic and used her busyness to avoid feelings that she didn't want to face up to. No wonder she was, as she said, "too uptight to relax" with her husband. So she taught him how to relax her feet with reflexology techniques, and immediately her entire body relaxed into the mood she needed. Reflexology literally made feet first in their foreplay rituals!

GOOD STEPS: FOR SEXUAL DYSFUNCTION

Each session should last 30 minutes and be given 2 or 3 times a week, especially when both of you can relax and enjoy being together.

1. Relax both feet with relaxation techniques, and end by a thumb press on the solar plexus point in both feet. Relax each foot separately.

2. Thumb walk up the five zones of one foot and work the points suggested below.

3. Thumb walk up the fives zones of the other foot and work the points suggested below.

4. Integrate relaxation techniques throughout the session as needed to help your partner relax when you encounter tender spots.

REFLEX AREA	TECHNIQUE	RATIONALE
CHEST/LUNG/BREAST REGION	Thumb walk	• Regulate and normalize breathing and heart functions
DIAPHRAGM	Rotate onto thumb	• Free blocked emotions
LUNGS AND CHEST	Lung press	• Relax chest • Deepen breathing
THYROID	Thumb walk	• Balance energy • Produce hormones for development of nervous system
BRAIN	Finger roll	• Relax mind • Soothe nerve impulses for better sexual response
SPINE	Spinal twist	• Stretch spine
SPINE	Thumb walk up, down, and across	• Balance the nervous system • Improve nerve flow to sexual organs
CHRONIC AREA/HIP	Finger walk	• Improve energy and blood flow to sexual organs
GROIN, FALLOPIAN TUBES, AND SEMINAL VESICLES	Ankle rotation	• Stimulate groin, fallopian tubes, and seminal vesicles
UTERUS/PROSTATE	Rotate onto finger	• Improve circulation and energy flow to sexual organs
OVARIES/TESTICLES	Small circular finger rotations	• Improve circulation and energy flow to sexual organs
ADRENALS	Rotate onto thumb	• Revitalize the body
ENTIRE FOOT	Wringing	• Relax entire foot and body
ENTIRE FOOT	Karate chops	• Get blood flowing

• Do relaxation techniques and thumb press on the solar plexus point in both feet, and end with breeze strokes.

Suggested Visualization:

Have your partner imagine herself in a very safe place—perhaps a bower of flowering trees deep in the forest, or a very special room of her own choosing. Have her open and close the door to the room (or the entrance to the scene) until she is convinced that she is totally protected. Then, let her imagine bringing her partner into the safe place and sharing a favorite form of sexual communication there, filled with light and love.

HEADACHES, ILLNESS, AND FATIGUE

In the traditional wedding vows, couples pledge to love each other "in sickness and in health." Naturally, most young, healthy brides and grooms are not seriously thinking about what could go wrong in this department when they marry. But the honeymoon of perfect health doesn't last forever! Before the year is out one of you will have had at least a cold. Hopefully, more serious illnesses do not strike, but in whatever way you make or interpret this vow, you are promising to take care of each other; and as you will soon discover, your mate's illness is also your own.

By practicing reflexology while you are still in good health, you also develop the habit of respecting and trusting each other as healers, as partners committed to providing a nurturing environment for each other. And of course, reflexology allows the body to relax, and only a relaxed body can heal itself. What's more, if the illness lasts for an extended period of time, the healthy partner will have to assume more of the responsibilities of running the household. Reflexology on yourself during these periods can make that burden more bearable.

One of my associates used reflexology on her husband when he was suffering agonizing migraines due to eyestrain and other physical and emotional problems. The headaches were so bad they feared a trip to the hospital was unavoidable. He took medication and she used reflexology on him while waiting for the medicine to take effect. Not only were the symptoms quickly relieved, but the fear surrounding the condition was alleviated and a trip to the emergency ward was unnecessary.

Statistically, couples have the advantage over single people when it comes to staying healthy. Undoubtedly part of this is due to being loved and cared for. Positive emotions are as important as chicken soup for getting well and staying well. It's also a blessing to know that in sickness and in health you are not alone. You have someone to share with. Even an illness becomes a shared event.

A major sexual disease of our times is herpes, a stress-related problem that can interfere with lovemaking. Herpes is most contagious when it flares up, and thousands of people afflicted with herpes lead safe, happy sexual lives by abstaining from sex when they break out with symptoms. Unfortunately, many people lead stressful lives, and worrying about herpes increases the stress all the more. Whereas some people show symptoms only a couple of times a year, others have them much more frequently and their sexual spontaneity suffers. At the present there is no cure for herpes, but if physical and emotional relaxation is a preventive therapy for flare-ups, reflexology can be the prescription for a more rewarding sex life.

Reflexology is also a great substitute in those periods when you are too tired for sex or can't find time for it. When you are young it's hard to imagine not being able to find time or energy for sex. Other people have trouble, but certainly not you, right? Wrong. Every couple's sexual life goes through patterns, ups and downs, periods when there is lots of sex interspersed with periods of little sex, periods of good sex and periods of not so good sex.

During the years when you're raising children, especially teenagers, you may find that your days and nights are totally taken up with them and their needs. What's more, these years often coincide with the peak years of your careers. It's no wonder that sex often ends up last on your list of things to do. Well, reflexology won't produce more hours in the day or night, but it can be a way to stay intimate with each other, relieve those proverbial "headaches," and give you a boost of energy so that you'll be more in the mood for making love. (It's up to you to find the time for it!) However you manage it, it's vitally important for the health of your relationship to stay intimate with each other during the good times and the bad times. "Intimate" means touching each other, and reflexology—like sex—is very hard to do without touching!

During periods of illness or fatigue when there doesn't seem to be time for sex, it's important to keep nurturing each other. Reflexology is a great way to do this and one that is equally available for men as well as women. In our society men are not encouraged to develop their nurturing talents to the fullest as women are, and yet they have them. Reflexology lets men play the nurturing role and experience this feminine aspect of their personalities in a positive way without feeling weak or emasculated. Too often men don't allow themselves to receive because they see that role as being too passive or submissive. It's part of the macho image that many men cultivate to be independent and always the giver, never the receiver. Reflexology can be the threshold for more complete development of the male psyche. It can introduce men to nurturing and to allowing themselves to receive nurturing in return.

GOOD STEPS: FOR NURTURING YOUR PARTNER

Do a full 30- to 50-minute session, interspersing relaxation techniques more lavishly than usual. Spend extra time on the relaxation and reflexology techniques that your partner finds particularly enjoyable.

Suggested Visualization:

As you work on your partner, imagine a beam or breeze of nourishing pink, green, gold, or lavender light (use whichever you like best) flowing from your heart and hands and enveloping his entire being. Ask your partner to see or feel this light enveloping him as you work. Try playing music that has special meaning for both of you during the session.

TALKING, SHARING, LISTENING

Communication is a must for a stable relationship. I firmly believe what so many couples' therapists point out—that most of the problems between two people are due to lack of communication or miscommunication. Reflexology is not an "open line," but just as it opens up parts of the body to allow energy to flow more smoothly, it also opens people up on deeper personal levels. When we are relaxed and worry-free, we feel more self-confident in expressing ourselves. Things we've kept bottled up because of feelings of insecurity can finally be spoken. We become more verbal.

Even in a professional setting, I find many of my clients want to unburden themselves as if I were their psychotherapist or counselor. They trust the safe environment that reflexology creates and they just open up and spill out their troubles. In fact, my husband, who *is* a psychotherapist, will often recommend that his clients see me first before they meet with him. This has proven so successful that even some of his own colleagues now send me their clients who are too stressed-out or uptight to make the most of a counseling session. After a reflexology session, they can go to their counseling sessions relaxed and ready to talk. If reflexology facilitates communication between people on a professional level, think of how it can build up feelings of trust and closeness between two people who love each other.

GOOD STEPS: FOR TALKING OVER SERIOUS ISSUES

Before beginning any serious discussion, especially on topics that you and your partner have differing views on, spend a half hour or so doing reflexology on each other. This need not be a full session. Relaxation techniques are often enough. You will find that the extra half hour actually shortens the amount of time the two of you need to talk since you will both be more open, relaxed and clearheaded.

Suggested Visualization:

Let your partner imagine she is sitting with you in a beautiful blue room with a wonderful view, working everything out.

MAKING DECISIONS TOGETHER

Communication skills are important in decision making. So many decisions can only be made successfully when both parties concur and feel their interests have been heard. Important decisions about such issues as finances, children, aging parents, and career changes require long hours of talking things over and weighing alternatives, setting goals and objectives, planning ahead. You are no longer just deciding for yourself. You have your "other half" to consider, and possibly children.

Decision making can be tough, but clearheadedness and the ability to put distractions aside can help, and reflexology can facilitate both. In fact, creativity studies have indicated that some of our best ideas and insights come when we are in an alpha state, that state of consciousness when the brain produces alpha waves. It happens when we daydream or meditate, perform some simple repetitive task, or just let thoughts flow freely. It doesn't come when we are pressured, distracted, or trying to meet deadlines.

I can't guarantee that reflexology will assure that you make the right decisions, but I can assure you that decision making will be easier in the deep, relaxing alpha state of consciousness that reflexology produces. Many of my clients who are top executives claim that they get more things decided after their weekly sessions than they do stewing at their desks. Furthermore, people tend to sleep better after reflexology, and we all know how a good night's sleep can put worries and problems into perspective so that we can think about them more clearly.

Most couples go through a lot of serious decision making during their midlife crises. Somewhere in their late thirties or early forties men and women begin to reexamine themselves and ask if they want to spend the second half of their lives doing the same things, living in the same ways, shooting for the same goals. They may experience the "last chance syndrome" —make the move now because you aren't getting any younger. It's during this time that many people switch careers or get divorced. Obviously, serious decisions such as these should not be made hastily or out of desperation. You need time to relax, get unstressed, and make your decision from a calm center.

Often the mid-life crisis is characterized by depression and anxiety, and too many people resort to drugs or alcohol to cope with it. Or they go under a doctor's care and use prescription drugs to see them through. Many of my clients say that reflexology has made a great difference in the way they handle their mid-life crises. They look forward to their weekly session, which sends them back to their lives renewed, relaxed, feeling better about themselves, and I hope more clearheaded and committed to making the best choices for themselves and the ones they love.

It's also around this time that many marriages get shaken up because of the "empty nest syndrome." The kids leave home. For some couples, this is just what they have been waiting for! I don't mean this in a cynical sense. Marriage counselors agree that human beings are not meant to be live-in parents all life long! Parenting is only one stage in the passages of our lives, a stage that must come to an end. At some point children go off to lead their own lives, and every couple must learn how to live alone again and make crucial decisions about how they want to spend the rest of their lives.

One of my clients went through a deep period of depression after the last of her four children left home. The two older boys had left the nest several years before; but her two daughters, about four years apart in age, both left home within a couple of months of each other. My client had not expected that they would leave together and so soon. She had counted on the youngest child's living at home for a while. But as fate would have it, the girl received a scholarship to a college out of state. The mother took it rather hard and came to me to begin reflexology for this very reason. After a few sessions, she began to handle her changed home life much better and decided to enroll in my training program. Soon she began an informal reflexology career for herself and found that in this way she could continue her role as caretaker and nurturer, something that had been the heart of her life as a mother.

Some couples look forward to this passage in life. Others dread it, especially women whose lives and identities centered around being mothers. It's at these times that a couple must look to each other for support and companionship in order to turn their bustling household into a quiet home that the two of them share, as they once did when they were young and just starting out. Reflexology can be the vehicle that helps them through the transition.

REFLEXOLOGY FOR ENDING ARGUMENTS

Reflexology can also be a great way to end arguments. It's always been part of the folklore that making up is the best part of an argument. The truth of the matter is that it's often hard to initiate lovemaking when we feel like killing each other. But it's not so hard to grab a foot! In fact, some successfully married couples use personal rituals to end arguments or to stop talking about a touchy subject for the moment. Reflexology can be that ritual. Literally, take a foot and start in. You don't even have to say, "I'm sorry." Your hands say it for you. What frequently happens is that as you relax and calm down, you can see things more clearly and get the situation in better perspective. Sometimes we discover that we really aren't angry at our mates; they were simply the handiest targets for relieving stress.

GOOD STEPS: FOR ENDING ARGUMENTS

Sit on the floor or a firm bed, facing each other so that you can each reach the other's feet. One person's leg will lie inside the other's.

Hold the solar plexus point on both feet for about 2 minutes, increasing and decreasing the amount of pressure with your thumbs every few seconds. Continue with a lengthy period of relaxation techniques, occasionally running your thumb from the heel up to the solar plexus point and hold it for a moment.

A full session is not necessary.

Agree ahead of time that you will not talk to each other until after the session. Most important, agree not to talk about whatever it was you were arguing about when you began!

While holding the solar plexus point, breathe together. Focus on the exhalation, consciously releasing the anger as you breathe out.

REFLEX AREA	TECHNIQUE	RATIONALE
DIAPHRAGM	Rotate onto thumb and thumb walk across	• Open breathing to help relax
LUNGS AND CHEST	Lung press	• Reduce stress
ENTIRE FOOT	Thumb slide, thumb rotations	• Relaxation
ADRENALS	Rotate onto thumb	• Balance adrenaline level
ENTIRE FOOT	Karate chops, punch, slap	• Release built-up energy

Suggested Visualization:

Let your partner see the exhalations of breath as red flames of anger being released from the inside. Encourage him to see the flames dispersing into the air. Then, let your partner imagine he is breathing in the scent of beautiful, cool flowers in an English garden after the rain. After a few minutes (or whenever seems right) ask your partner to imagine the two of you together in the garden, setting up a picnic of your favorite foods.

Do this visualization along with your partner while you give the session, and let him know that you are doing it, too.

THE BALANCE OF POWER

Every relationship is in some ways a power relationship, and that in itself can cause problems, especially if one partner wields too much power. In the most stable relationships, power is shared or balanced out in that each party exercises authority in distinct and agreed-upon areas.

In traditional marriages, of course, the husband was the breadwinner and took care of things like the car; the wife was in charge of domestic concerns and the kids. In many modern marriages, and especially in live-in relationships, these roles get divvied up differently based on time, interest, and the natural talents of the two people. Nevertheless, power is always shifting. It is never completely stabilized, and often one or the other may begin to feel too submissive and grow resentful.

A couple who practice mutual reflexology have a good buffer to the "power game." In reflexology each party plays both roles: giver and receiver, dominant and submissive, healer and heal-ee. There's no better activity for eliminating competition. Reflexology is the great equalizer. No matter who is better at career, cooking, getting along with the children, or tinkering with the car, in the quiet hours of reflexology they are truly partners and equals.

GOOD STEPS: FOR FEELING LIKE EQUALS

Sit facing each other on a firm bed or the floor as described in the Good Steps for Ending an Argument (p. 165).

Treat each other to a long session of relaxation techniques and then move on to work all areas of the foot with regular reflexology.

Always work the same foot on each other. Both of you should work the same points, with one partner setting the order on the first foot and the other partner setting the order on the second foot. A reflexology game of follow-the-leader!

Suggested Visualization:

Let your partner imagine you are with her together in a fantastic amusement park (or hiking along a breathtaking nature trail, or walking through a wonderful exhibit in your favorite museum), enjoying all the rides together.

Reflexology is truly an act of love. People who receive reflexology speak about it in terms of love, and reflexologists themselves (even professional ones) know that the best sessions are given in love. I can't emphasize enough that the intention of the reflexologist is paramount in the healing process. In fact, I believe that a strong love between two people will more than compensate for lack of experience in reflexology, and that years of experience in reflexology alone without the love leaves a lot to be desired.

People who love each other are twice blessed: Not only is there someone who loves them, there is someone who will take care of them. Reflexology can be an exciting part of both the caring and the loving.

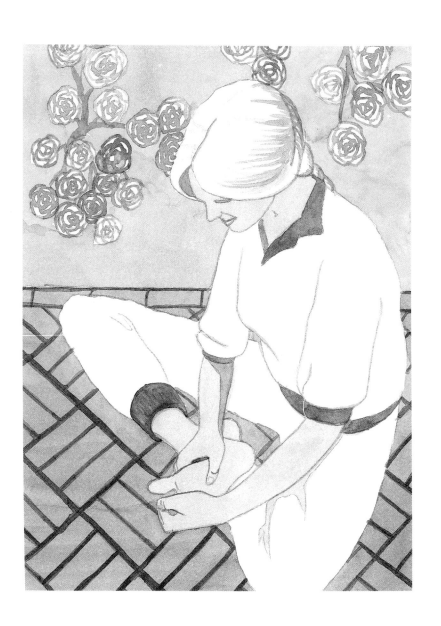

CHAPTER SEVEN

THE CYCLES OF LIFE:

REFLEXOLOGY FOR WOMEN

The roles women fill in society have changed greatly over the last generation. For some women the changes have been welcome and long overdue;
others wish they had never occurred. I'm hard pressed to think of a women I
know, either a traditional wife and mother, a single career woman, or a
woman trying to combine both, who is not frequently under a lot of stress,
confronted with issues and responsibilities our mothers and grandmothers
never had to face. It's easy to lose touch with ourselves in such a challenging
world. As women we owe it to ourselves to take time to meet our special
needs whatever walk of life we are in. We need to let go and indulge ourselves
in activities of self-nurturing and self-acceptance. We need to relax and renew
our energies so that we can come back to our duties and responsibilities
balanced, clearheaded, and capable of doing our best.

Speaking for myself personally and for the many women clients I have
known over the years, reflexology is a perfect way for a woman to take time
out to relax, to be nurtured, to find her own interior sense of worth. I have
watched reflexology help many women from all types of backgrounds and
with all kinds of problems. No matter why they come to us, our clients attest
to the fact that reflexology relaxes them, assists their bodies in healing, balances them, and helps them put problems in perspective so they can handle
them realistically and effectively.

SKIN CARE

Today both women and men take great pains to improve their complexions.
It's hard to say who are more vain! Cosmetics and skin care products for both
sexes are a multimillion-dollar business. For generations women have been
"fixing their make-up and powdering their noses" to please men and themselves. Even today with the emphasis on more "natural" looks and less make-
up, women are still concerned that their skin stay young and healthy-looking.
While everyone's skin is destined to eventually look older—there's not much
that can be done about it—there is a lot that can be done to keep it both
healthy and healthy-looking.

My clients who look at themselves in the mirror after a session are always
pleased at how good they look. Dark circles and puffiness under the eyes
disappear or fade. Tension lines and general tiredness are gone. The tightness
in the jawline that indicates determination and rigidity softens. Usually the

skin glows. And the reason has nothing to do with magic or miracles. It's really quite simple: a relaxed face looks more beautiful; and when circulation is improved, the skin takes on a healthy glow. Our faces—eyes, mouths, skin —express the physical tension in our bodies, as well as our worries and negative feelings. Reflexology relaxes the entire body and mind. Once the tension is released the face shows it.

Recovering from plastic surgery is a very uncomfortable ordeal, but one woman who began reflexology with one of my associates the very day after surgery healed in half the normal time. Her doctor had never seen such quick recovery before and concluded that it was the regular relaxation, improved circulation, and general balancing of bodily functions that pulled her through the recovery period so quickly and with relatively little pain.

Remember: before each routine in this chapter, set up the environment as described in Chapter Three. Prepare the materials needed, such as lotion, towel, and cornstarch. Create the appropriate mood with lighting and music. Review the person's health history. Check the feet for cuts, bruises, sores, corns, or calluses. If necessary, clean the feet with a warm washcloth or handiwipe. Clear and center yourself.

GOOD STEPS: FOR ACNE AND SKIN DISORDERS

Many skin disorders are due to stress and excess toxins, so a reflexology session that works the liver, kidneys, urinary system, and intestines could be beneficial.

Each session should last 15 minutes and be done 2 to 3 times a week.

1. Relax both feet with relaxation techniques, and end by a thumb press on the solar plexus point in both feet. Relax each foot separately.

2. Thumb walk up the five zones of one foot and work the points suggested below.

3. Thumb walk up the five zones of the other foot and work the points suggested below.

4. Integrate relaxation techniques throughout the session as needed to help your partner relax when you encounter tender spots.

REFLEX AREA	TECHNIQUE	RATIONALE
THYROID AT BASE OF BIG TOE	Thumb walk across	• Regulate metabolism of skin cells • Affects overall skin health
THYROID FRONT OF BASE OF BIG TOE	Finger walk across	• Regulate metabolism of skin cells
LYMPHATICS/NECK, CHEST	Finger walk	• Help waste elimination
PITUITARY	Hook & back-up	• Regulate all hormonal activity
DIAPHRAGM TO PELVIC LINE WITH EMPHASIS ON LIVER	Thumb walk and pivot on diagonal, crosshatching	• Improve waste elimination
KIDNEYS	Rotate onto thumb	• Help in waste elimination
ADRENALS	Rotate onto thumb	• Fight inflammation and produce cortisone • Water and mineral balance

•   Do relaxation techniques and thumb press on the solar plexus point in both feet, and end with breeze strokes.

Suggested Visualization:

Let your partner imagine she is in a quiet place (perhaps her favorite natural setting) listening to the wind or to a babbling brook. Have her see herself with clear, beautiful skin in this setting. If she likes, she can imagine a close friend or loved one approaching and embracing her.

MENSTRUAL PROBLEMS

Many women become more regular in their menstrual cycles with reflexology. The chemical changes that occur each month evoke real physical and emotional discomfort. For a few days, the body is not in its normal hormonal balance. The result can be mood swings, irritability, and physical discomfort from cramps, headaches and tender breasts.

The phenomenon of menstrual cramping is a result of uterine smooth-muscle contractions, but the amount of pain experienced seems to be related to calcium levels in the blood, among other things. Tender breasts are caused in part by hormones and fluid retention, and possibly by the presence of certain toxins, like caffeine, in the blood. Fluid retention and calcium levels can be affected through work on the kidney, thyroid, and parathyroid reflex areas.

There has been much discussion lately over premenstrual syndrome (PMS). Several of my female clients suffering from severe PMS discovered that with regular reflexology sessions the days leading up to their monthly periods became calmer and they found it easier to stay in control.

One woman who came to me for reflexology was approaching menopause and had missed her period for four or five months. She wondered if this was the real thing since she hadn't expected her "change of life" to begin for at least a few more years. She had just one session and later that day her period began. Several clients who have missed periods and suspected they were pregnant (but were not) began to ovulate shortly after I worked on the areas for the reproductive organs. In its subtle and gentle way, reflexology balances the abnormalities that cause their periods to be late.

There are many reasons why women are not regular or miss periods, some of them biochemical, others stress-related. In general, reflexology has been a boon in getting many women back on more regular cycles.

GOOD STEPS: FOR REGULATING MENSTRUATION

Begin sessions the week before menstruation and continue once a day during menstruation. Each session should last 15 minutes.

1. Relax both feet with relaxation techniques, and end by a thumb press on the solar plexus point in both feet. Relax each foot separately.

2. Thumb walk up the five zones of one foot and work the points suggested below.

3. Thumb walk up the five zones of the other foot and work the points suggested below.

4.   Integrate relaxation techniques throughout the session as needed to help your partner relax when you encounter tender spots.

REFLEX AREA	TECHNIQUE	RATIONALE
CHEST, LUNG AND BREAST AREA	Thumb walk	• Regulate breathing • Relax muscles • Oxygenate cells
DIAPHRAGM	Rotate onto thumb	• Regulate breathing • Relax muscles • Oxygenate cells
THYROID AND PARATHYROIDS	Thumb walk across	• Regulate calcium levels
BRAIN	Finger roll	• Relieve pressure and fluid accumulation in brain
PITUITARY	Hook & back-up	• Stimulate the endocrine system • Help defend against cystic breasts
SPINE	Thumb walk up and down	• Relieve back strain and cramps by increased flow to pelvic region
LIVER	Thumb walk	• Detoxify blood • Formation of blood constituents
PANCREAS	Thumb walk across	• Balance blood sugars
KIDNEYS	Rotate onto thumb	• Eliminate fluid retention
ADRENALS	Rotate onto thumb	• Regulate mineral balance • Renew energy • Release hydrocortisone, which reduces swelling
INTESTINES	Thumb walk	• Balance to aid constipation or diarrhea
OVARIES	Small circular finger rotations	• Stimulate production of estrogens and progesterones
UTERUS	Rotate onto finger and finger walk	• Improve circulation and cleanse uterine walls
FALLOPIAN TUBES	Finger walk across	• Maintain clear passage from ovaries to uterus

- Do relaxation techniques and thumb press on the solar plexus point in both feet, and end with breeze strokes.

Suggested Visualization:

Let your partner imagine soft, cool ocean waves massaging her entire body and restoring her to her own perfect rhythm as you work.

MENOPAUSE

During menopause (technically, the cessation of menses for a complete year) a woman is susceptible to hot flashes and increased perspiration. These are physical conditions directly related to the hormonal changes taking place in her body. As you know, however, some women undergo a whole list of other physical symptoms which most gynecologists will agree are produced by stress, worry, and other changes in the woman's lifestyle that usually occur at this time rather than the hormonal changes. Reflexology can make these changes more bearable and relieve the stress and tension that cause so many side effects.

GOOD STEPS: FOR MENOPAUSE

Each session should last 20 to 30 minutes and be given twice a week.

1. Relax both feet with relaxation techniques, and end by a thumb press on the solar plexus point in both feet. Relax each foot separately.

2. Thumb walk up the five zones of one foot and work the points suggested below.

3. Thumb walk up the five zones of the other foot and work the points suggested below.

4. Integrate relaxation techniques throughout the session as needed to help your partner relax when you encounter tender spots.

REFLEX AREA	TECHNIQUE	RATIONALE
THYROID AND PARATHYROIDS	Thumb walk across	• Normalize calcium and phosphorus levels in the bone
HELPER AREA TO THYROID	Thumb walk	• Release hormones which help in dealing with stress
BRAIN	Finger roll	• Control the emotional and physical balance of the body
PITUITARY	Hook & back-up	• Regulate endocrine glands • Help control hot flashes
HYPOTHALAMUS	Hook & back-up	• Control body temperature
LIVER	Thumb walk on a diagonal	• Source of body heat
KIDNEYS	Rotate onto thumb	• Filter and cleanse blood • Balance water
ADRENALS	Rotate onto thumb	• Energy balancing • Cortex produces sex hormones
HIP TRIANGLE	Finger walk	• Help circulation to reproductive area
UTERUS	Press third finger and rotate onto point	• Maintain circulation to uterus
OVARIES	Small circular finger rotations	• Regulate estrogen level
FALLOPIAN TUBE	Over-ankle rotation	• Stimulate and relax area to the fallopian tube
ACHILLES TENDON	Finger walk up sides of ankle	• Circulation to reproductive organs and sciatic nerve
UTERUS, CHRONIC AREA	Thumb walk down	• Improve energy and circulation

• Do relaxation techniques and thumb press on the solar plexus point in both feet, and end with breeze strokes.

Suggested Visualization:

Let your partner imagine she is piloting a gorgeous red and orange hot-air balloon over a countryside of castles and rivers, with her own partner by her side. Have her imagine herself navigating all the air currents with perfect mastery and serenity, until she finally lands the balloon gently in a field, and she and her loved one hop out for a champagne picnic in a garden of fragrant honeysuckle.

CANCER

Breast and cervical cancer can cause panic and anxiety, but the emotional repercussions can often be tempered by reflexology. In addition to worry over the physical dangers and possible need for surgery, a woman's self-image is badly shaken by these disorders that portend the possibility of a hysterectomy or mastectomy. We know that alternative therapies such as visualization and affirmations, along with a formal program of counseling and relaxation, have caused cancer to go into remission in some people. The general effect of these activities is to strengthen the immune system.

If surgery is necessary, recovery can be long and painful. Both the body and the self-image need to repair. Reflexology can speed up the time needed to recover from major surgery and make the recovery process itself more bearable.

GOOD STEPS: FOR OVARIAN/BREAST CYSTS OR GROWTHS

Each session should last 20 minutes and be given 3 or 4 times a week.

1. Relax both feet with relaxation techniques, and end by a thumb press on the solar plexus point in both feet. Relax each foot separately.

2. Thumb walk up the five zones of one foot and work the points suggested below.

3. Thumb walk up the five zones of the other foot and work the points suggested below.

4. Integrate relaxation techniques throughout the session as needed to help your partner relax when you encounter tender spots.

REFLEX AREA	TECHNIQUE	RATIONALE
LUNGS AND CHEST	Thumb walk zones	• Improve circulation
LUNGS AND CHEST	Lung press	• Relax chest region • Ease breathing
LYMPHATICS IN BREAST AREA	Finger walk	• Release fluids
THYROID	Thumb walk	• Metabolic functions
PITUITARY	Hook & back-up	• Balance endocrine functions and growth of cells
SPINE (THORACIC 1–7)	Thumb walk	• Improve blood and nerve flow to breast region
SPLEEN	Rotate onto thumb and thumb walk	• Increase immune function
LIVER	Thumb walk on diagonal	• Filter wastes from the body to improve detoxification function
BLADDER, KIDNEYS	Rotate onto thumb	• Filter/cleanse blood
URETERS	Thumb walk up	• Release blockage
OVARIES	Finger walk	• Balance hormone release
UTERUS	Rotate onto finger and finger walk	• Improve circulation and energy flow
LYMPHATICS IN GROIN	Over ankle rotations	• Drainage

•   Do relaxation techniques and thumb press on the solar plexus point in both feet, and end with breeze strokes.

Suggested Visualization:

Have your partner visualize her cyst or growth as a pink knot, and then have her untie the knot until it is unfolded into a beautiful, loose, shimmering piece of pink fabric she can make into anything she wants.

OSTEOPOROSIS

Recently, much media attention has been paid to a condition associated with aging called osteoporosis. Osteoporosis is a condition of porousness in bone that causes spontaneous fractures, loss of height, and a deformity called the "dowager's hump." While both men and women can be affected, osteoporosis occurs twice as often in women for several reasons, primarily: 1) the cessation of estrogen production in postmenopausal women and 2) a woman's increased calcium requirement during pregnancy and nursing. In addition, our sedentary lifestyles and generally calcium-poor diets contribute to this condition in later life.

While reflexology is no substitute for correcting dietary intake of calcium, for exercise, or for the delicate hormonal balance which is required for calcium absorption from the diet into the bones, reflexology will increase circulation and vitality and aid in digestion of all nutrients.

GOOD STEPS: FOR OSTEOPOROSIS

Each session should last 15 to 20 minutes and be given twice a week.

1. Relax both feet with relaxation techniques, and end by a thumb press on the solar plexus point in both feet. Relax each foot separately.

2. Thumb walk up the five zones of one foot and work the points suggested below.

3. Thumb walk up the five zones of the other foot and work the points suggested below.

4. Integrate relaxation techniques throughout the session as needed to help your partner relax when you encounter tender spots.

REFLEX AREA	TECHNIQUE	RATIONALE
NECK, THYROID AND PARATHYROIDS	Thumb walk across	• Activate endocrine system • Balance calcium levels
PITUITARY	Hook & back-up	• Stimulate all endocrine glands
SPINE	Spinal twist	• Stretch spine
SPINE	Thumb walk up, down, across, and rotate onto thumb	• Improve nerve response in skeletal system
HIP/KNEE/LEG REFLEX AREA	Finger walk	• Relieve stress • Increase circulation in these commonly afflicted areas
SPLEEN	Rotate onto thumb	• Activate immune system
LIVER	Thumb walk diagonally	• Detoxification of blood • Formation of blood constituents
ADRENALS	Rotate onto thumb and pivot	• Cortex produces estrogen • Reduce inflammation • Control sodium, potassium, and water balance
OVARIES	Finger walk	• Estrogen release
ENTIRE FOOT	Wringing	• Relax entire foot and body
POINTS THAT CORRESPOND TO AFFLICTED AREA	Work	• Stimulate healing activity directly in afflicted areas

•   Do relaxation techniques and thumb press on the solar plexus point in both feet, and end with breeze strokes.

Suggested Visualization:

Let your partner imagine she is in the center of a circle of her loved ones, who are listening to her confide her innermost thoughts or feelings. Ask her to imagine soft white beams of light holding her and supporting her. Then ask her to feel all the hands of her loved ones holding her straight and firm and tall.

PREGNANCY

Pregnancy is an important event in the lives of women and their mates. Women don't become mothers alone, and becoming a father has its own unique complications. Let's consider in some detail the many benefits that reflexology can bring to you, your mate, and the unborn child.

Infertility

The first problem that some couples face is *getting* pregnant! When a doctor tells a woman who has difficulty conceiving that "it's all in your head," I always say, "Well, if the problem's in the head, the solution is partially in your feet!" Reflexology can offer a way out of this perplexing dilemma. If there is a genuine physical problem, such as a disorder in the reproductive system, a woman should follow the advice of her gynecologist. But when you are told that "there's nothing wrong *physically*," that your problem is primarily psychological, what can you do? Psychological problems always seem more elusive and harder to pin down than physical ones. Additional worry about being infertile only compounds the situation, and the diagnosis becomes self-fulfilling. It becomes a marital Catch-22. You can't get pregnant until you relax and you can't relax because you're worried that you can't get pregnant. Worry and anxiety over not being able to have children can create the very physical conditions that prevent conception.

The nonphysical causes of infertility lie in the unnecessary stress and anxiety that grow out of many legitimate concerns, such as the relationship with your husband, the responsibility that having children will bring, the changes in your job or career, even the degree of sexual satisfaction in your marital relationship. Just the thought of becoming pregnant and becoming a mother can cause tension on a subconscious level even if you aren't totally aware of it.

Deep relaxation alleviates stress and tension so that conception may take place. When the husband gives reflexology to his wife, the married couple experiences a growing closeness and warmth that in itself can build the trust and assurance a woman may need to be physically receptive. Not only are reflexology sessions relaxing and enjoyable, but the released energy gently stimulates the reproductive organs and promotes normal glandular functioning.

GOOD STEPS: FOR OVERCOMING INFERTILITY

Each session should last 20 to 30 minutes. Begin sessions a couple of days before ovulation; continue each day during ovulation and for a couple of days afterward. Also for general care, continue sessions twice a week throughout the month.

1.   Relax both feet with relaxation techniques, and end by a thumb press on the solar plexus point in both feet. Relax each foot separately.

2.   Thumb walk up the five zones of one foot and work the points suggested below.

3.   Thumb walk up the five zones of the other foot and work the points suggested below.

4.   Integrate relaxation techniques throughout the session as needed to help your partner relax when you encounter tender spots.

REFLEX AREA	TECHNIQUE	RATIONALE
THYROID	Thumb walk across	• Regulate metabolic rate
TOP OF FOOT	Vibrate fingers down	• Relaxation
PITUITARY	Hook & back-up	• Improve hormonal environment for conception
SPINE	Spinal twist	• Loosen spine • Improve circulation
LUMBARS	Thumb walk down and across and rotate into thumb	• Stimulate nerves to pelvic area • Balance nervous system, resulting in more relaxed emotional state
ENTIRE FOOT	Wringing	• Relax entire foot and body
ADRENALS	Rotate onto thumb	• Heighten energy • Cortex produces sex hormones

REPRODUCTIVE AREAS CHRONIC	Finger walk	• Encourage secretion of reproductive hormones
UTERUS/PROSTATE	Rotate onto finger	• Enrich blood supply to reproductive organs and glands
OVARIES/TESTICLES	Small circular finger rotations	• Encourage secretion of sex hormones
REPRODUCTIVE ORGANS AND GLANDS	Ankle boogie	• Stimulate reproductive organs
FALLOPIAN TUBES/ SEMINAL VESICLES	Finger walk across	• Relieve obstruction or blockages to conception
FALLOPIAN TUBES/ SEMINAL VESICLES	Over ankle rotation	• Stimulate groin, fallopian tubes, seminal vesicles
ENTIRE FOOT	Foot boogie	• Relax entire foot and body

• Do relaxation techniques and thumb press on the solar plexus point in both feet, and end with breeze strokes.

Suggested Visualization:

Let your partner imagine and feel a beautiful, fragrant red rose unfolding at the base of his or her spine. If your partner is a woman, once the rose is in place, have her imagine it multiplying into a profusion of beautiful deep red roses that softly fill her womb. If your partner is a man, have him imagine the rose growing outward until it touches his partner, and covers her with roses.

Common Ailments During Pregnancy

Nature never intended pregnancy to be a form of disease, and yet some women experience it as a long period of discomfort and fatigue. From the initial bouts of morning sickness after conception to the physical discomforts in the reproductive organs after delivery, having a baby is physically stressful and for some women an annoying ordeal. It doesn't have to be. The fact that a good number of women have relatively painless and easy pregnancies is strong evidence that when the body processes function properly, having children can be one of life's greatest joys, not a major source of aggravation.

Yet there's no getting around it: bringing a new life into the world is not a simple matter. It's not easy providing for your own life as well as for that of your child. Even in the first few months of existence, an unborn baby uses enormous amounts of nutrients that would ordinarily go to providing energy for the mother in her normal activities. But not only are her activities not normal, mom-to-be has less energy to go around. It is the first indication to the new mother that her life from now on will be one of sharing, including the energy sources needed even more at this critical time when daily activities become increasingly fatiguing.

There can also be complications. The list of potential physical ailments for the pregnant woman can look forboding to someone who doesn't realize that many of them can be avoided or minimized by proper treatment. In fact, reflexology has something to offer in the way of relief for each, and in some cases, instant relief. The most common problems—most of which are listed in the table of common conditions in Chapter Fifteen—include back strain, constipation, dizziness, fluid retention, general fatigue, headache, hemorrhoids, hypertension, insomnia, leg cramps, nausea, sore breasts, stomach cramps, and swollen ankles.

GOOD STEPS: DURING PREGNANCY

Each session should last 30 minutes and be given 2 or 3 times a week or whenever feeling discomfort. During the first and third trimester of pregnancy, gently work the ankles. Work the chronic area during second trimester.

1.   Relax both feet with relaxation techniques, and end by a thumb press on the solar plexus point in both feet. Relax each foot separately.

2.   Thumb walk up the five zones of one foot and work the points suggested below.

3.   Thumb walk up the five zones of the other foot and work the points suggested below.

4.   Integrate relaxation techniques throughout the session as needed to help your partner relax when you encounter tender spots.

REFLEX AREA	TECHNIQUE	RATIONALE
CHEST	Thumb walk	• Relax and deepen breathing
LUNG AND CHEST	Lung press	• Relax chest area
BREAST AND MAMMARY GLANDS	Finger walk	• Decrease sensitivity in area
THYROID, PARATHYROIDS, AND AREAS RELATIVE TO THE THYROID	Thumb walk	• Balance metabolism and mineral levels • Responsible for growth and development
PITUITARY	Hook & back-up	• Improve nervous activity • Alleviate sluggishness
SPINE	Thumb walk up, down, and across	• Help circulation and nerve flow to spine
SPINE	Spinal twist	• Stretch spine
STOMACH	Thumb walk	• Discourage nausea by balancing stomach enzymes and acids
LIVER	Thumb walk on a diagonal, crosshatching	• Detoxification • Energy balance • Blood production • Improved portal circulation resulting in decreased leg swelling
ILEOCECAL VALVE	Hook & back-up	• Aid digestion and absorbtion
INTESTINES	Thumb walk	• Aid elimination and absorbtion
SIGMOID COLON	Thumb walk from bladder on 45° angle to zone 3½ Hook & back-up	• Aid movement of waste material into rectal area
SMALL INTESTINE	Thumb walk on a diagonal	• Improve peristaltic action
BLADDER AND KIDNEYS	Thumb walk	• Encourage elimination • Prevent fluid buildup

ADRENALS	Thumb walk and rotate onto thumb	• Balance energy levels • Improved muscle function for aid during labor and delivery
UTERUS	Rotate onto middle finger	• Circulation and energy flow
OVARIES	Small circular finger rotations	• Hormone production
FALLOPIAN TUBES	Finger walk	• Circulation • Energy flow
GROIN AND FALLOPIAN TUBES	Over-ankle rotation	• Stimulate groin and fallopian tubes
REPRODUCTIVE AREA	Ankle boogie	• Relax reproductive area
OVARIES AND UTERUS CHRONIC	Finger walk up	• Circulation • Energy flow
REPRODUCTIVE AREA	Thumb press	• Reduce swelling • Improve circulation to reproductive organs
UTERUS	Thumb walk down	
ENTIRE FOOT	Foot boogie	• Relax entire foot and body

• Do relaxation techniques and thumb press on the solar plexus point in both feet, and end with breeze strokes.

Suggested Visualization:

Have your partner see herself playing with a beautiful, healthy baby in the child's room.

In addition to the physical disorders that accompany a difficult pregnancy, there can be psychological problems as well. Having a baby is a stressful event. Becoming a mother is one of the major passages in a woman's life and preparing for it can cause worry—about the ways that pregnancy can disrupt your regular lifestyle, the health of the unborn child, how easy the delivery will be, the child's health after birth, and in general what life holds in store for you, your husband, and your new child. It's normal to wonder how your relationship with your husband will change as you both become parents in addition to being friends, companions, and lovers.

In working with both wives and husbands, I've found that the amount of worry varies from couple to couple, and that those who employ strategies to reduce the amount of stress generated by the pregnancy usually have fewer physical ailments. They sleep better, are less prone to colds, are not as irritable with each other, and are more sexually responsive. In short, they provide a healthier environment for themselves and the unborn baby, which reacts to the stress level of the mother even before it begins its own stressful life out in the world.

The Father's Role

Pregnant women have told me countless times how important it is for their husbands to join them in reflexology sessions during pregnancy. So often in the past we thought that being pregnant was a woman's job alone. Today we have more enlightened ideas about carrying and birthing a child. The father too experiences a disruption in his normal lifestyle when his wife is with child. Although men may not admit it, their own rite of passage in becoming fathers can be as worrisome as their wives. Fathers-to-be can feel cut off from their wives, who become more withdrawn and preoccupied with the female mysteries transpiring within their bodies. Eventually, normal sexual patterns will be interrupted and the couple must seek creative alternatives that are comfortable and satisfying for both of them. And the father can sink into his own worries—about his wife's health, about how much the new child will cost, about his need to take over some of his wife's duties while she is pregnant, including more of the child-rearing tasks if there are already other children. It's a time when a married couple should grow closer, but I've seen many grow more distant as each becomes more preoccupied with his or her own life.

Reflexology can provide times to be together in a loving and sensitive way; it can become part of the sensuous rituals that mean so much in expressing your love for each other. You'll discover that reflexology is both affectionate play and serious therapy. It can be a key to continuing communication, an important way to express your deepest desires to take care of each other.

GOOD STEPS: FOR COUPLES DURING PREGNANCY

See Good Steps for Lovemaking, page 154, and Good Steps for Nurturing, page 161, in Chapter Six.

LABOR

Both parents are now playing a major role in childbirth. In recent generations in the West, giving birth was considered a woman's responsibility, undertaken in the presence of a physician. Today fathers are playing important roles in the actual delivery of their babies, by participating in natural childbirth and by being in the delivery room to support and encourage the new mother. Reflexology can be a vital aspect of the labor process.

GOOD STEPS: DURING LABOR

Begin sessions when labor begins at home, continue in the hospital. Each session should last 10 to 15 minutes and be given every hour if possible.

1. Relax both feet with relaxation techniques, and end by a thumb press on the solar plexus point in both feet. Relax each foot separately.

2. Thumb walk up the five zones of one foot and work the points suggested below.

3. Thumb walk up the five zones of the other foot and work the points suggested below.

4. Integrate relaxation techniques throughout the session as needed to help your partner relax when you encounter tender spots.

REFLEX AREA	TECHNIQUE	RATIONALE
LUNGS AND CHEST	Thumb walk	• Regulate breathing
DIAPHRAGM	Thumb walk	• Relax breathing muscle • Improved deep breathing
BREAST	Finger walk	• Hormone production
SPINAL AREA (EMPHASIS ON LOWER SPINE)	Thumb walk up, down, and across	• Soothe neural activity • Release tension and pain in the lower back
SPINE	Spinal twist	• Stretch spine
SPINE	Rotate onto thumb	• Loosen spine and improve circulation
UTERUS	Rotate onto finger	• Improve blood flow and help in contractions
OVARIES	Small circular finger rotations	• Hormone production
ADRENALS	Rotate onto thumb	• Give energy for stamina

• Do relaxation techniques and thumb press on the solar plexus point in both feet, and end with breeze strokes.

Suggested Visualization:

Let your partner imagine she is resting in a comfortable, serene place with the baby in her arms.

AFTER THE BABY HAS ARRIVED

After the baby has arrived, the new mother has three primary goals, all of which can be expedited by regular home reflexology sessions. The first is to get her own body back into balance so that it returns to its regular metabolism. Specifically, the uterus has been stretched in pregnancy and childbirth and needs time to return to its normal condition. Working on the points that correspond to the reproductive organs will facilitate recovery by letting additional energy flow through those areas that need healing. Body weight should stabilize to what it was before pregnancy, and working the points for the thyroid, parathyroids, and pituitary will calm hunger and discourage overeating. In general, working the entire foot, with special emphasis on those parts that correspond to the trunk and limbs, will revitalize muscles and tone them up.

Secondly, if you breast-feed your baby, you should be ready for additional energy loss. Breast-feeding uses up considerable amounts of energy and nutrients. Some doctors estimate that it requires more energy to feed a baby than to carry it to term. Reflexology sessions working the points related to the breasts will aid in milk flow and minimize soreness. If you have previously been unable to nurse a baby because of lack of milk or overly sensitive breasts, you may discover after making reflexology part of your life that neither of these problems will recur. I've seen many women, convinced that they were not cut out to be breast-feeders because of experiences with previous babies, helped by reflexology—they find they can nurse a later baby and enjoy the close bonding that results.

Thirdly, you can begin early in applying reflexology techniques to your newborn's little feet. (See Chapter Eight.) No foot, no body is too small to benefit from reflexology. If your baby is colicky or cries a lot, working the point for the solar plexus will calm the little one down. Also, if the baby has trouble sleeping at night, stimulate the points for the diaphragm and all glands. When the child begins to teethe, work the areas at the base of the toenails.

GOOD STEPS: FOR POSTPARTUM RECOVERY

Each session should last 15 minutes and be given 2 or 3 times a week.

1.   Relax both feet with relaxation techniques, and end by a thumb press on the solar plexus point in both feet. Relax each foot separately.

2.   Thumb walk up the five zones of one foot and work the points suggested below.

3.   Thumb walk up the five zones of the other foot and work the points suggested below.

4.   Integrate relaxation techniques throughout the session as needed to help your partner relax when you encounter tender spots.

REFLEX AREA	TECHNIQUE	RATIONALE
CHEST AND DIAPHRAGM	Thumb walk	• Free breathing to help relax
MAMMARY GLANDS	Finger walk down	• Assist production of milk
BRAIN	Finger roll	• Regulate organs and glands and reduce emotional stress
PITUITARY	Hook & back-up	• Secrete hormones which affect emotional balance • Regulate glandular functions
KIDNEYS	Rotate onto thumb	• Normalize water level and reduce swelling
ADRENALS	Rotate onto thumb	• Boost energy • Produce hormones for mineral balance • Improve muscle tone
UTERUS	Rotate onto finger	• Maintain health and elasticity • Return to normal size and tone
OVARIES	Small circular finger rotations	• Regulate female hormones

•   Do relaxation techniques and thumb press on the solar plexus point in both feet, and end with breeze strokes.

Suggested Visualization:

Have your partner see herself as fit and energetic and partaking in a favorite prepregnancy activity (preferably one she has had to curtail or avoid during the pregnancy). Or, encourage her to see the pelvic area as a soft, pink silk sack, and have her imagine that sack lengthening and slimming into a beautiful, taut pink vase that contains whatever she likes.

Whatever lifestyle you pursue, take time out to make reflexology an integral part of it. You'll discover how being fit can be much more exhilarating than you ever imagined, and you'll be amazed at the energy and love you can bring to your relationships with children, spouse, colleagues, and friends. In other words, let reflexology help you be the best you can be.

CHAPTER EIGHT

GROWING FEET: CHILDREN'S REFLEXOLOGY

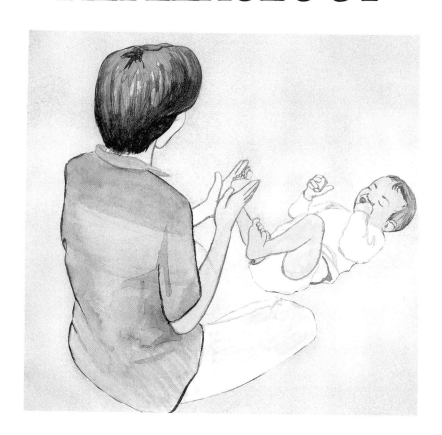

The world of children is not as carefree as adults might imagine. We can all recall the many joys and thrills of growing up, but there were also real growing pains too. And it's quite clear that not all of them were mumps, chicken pox, and broken bones. The childhood years can be filled with the psychological and emotional turmoil we usually think of as characteristic of adulthood. Children grow up very quickly today, facing issues and decisions both at home and school that would be stressful for even the most balanced adult. It is becoming common for young children to see psychiatrists, to experiment with drugs and alcohol in their teenage years, and to drop out of school and leave home before they are really ready to handle the outside world. Saddest of all, reports of teenage suicides are increasing. A Manhattan chiropractor told me that an alarming number of the children she sees professionally hold tension in their necks just like adults.

As parents we are concerned for our children's well-being. Our medicine cabinets are chock-full of remedies waiting for our children to show the first signs of colds or constipation or poison ivy. We know it's important to be prepared. Well, reflexology is like a home remedy kit and medicine cabinet all rolled into one. For both the physical ailments and psychological stresses of growing up, we should learn to reach for our children's feet as we do for children's aspirin. As preventive health care, reflexology may even make your family less reliant on the commercial products that promise health and well-being.

INTRODUCING CHILDREN TO REFLEXOLOGY

The first few months as a parent can become ever more joyful and meaningful as you get to know your child through reflexology. Those first critical months during which a newborn baby discovers the world outside the womb and learns to adapt to the realities of life can be the foundation for a strong relationship for both of you—a relationship that will continue throughout life. As you care for your baby in so many ways, the child learns to recognize you as the primary sources of comfort and warmth. Gently working the baby's foot provides pleasure and nurtures the bond between parent and child. By doing so, you'll assure a more stress-free infancy and your children will grow up with fond memories of how good it felt when mommy and daddy "played footsie" with them.

Generally, young children take very easily to reflexology. They like to give and receive; they have not built up many blocks and defenses about their bodies. They are not self-conscious. They enjoy being touched in playful ways. Reflexology also gives them a sense of security and nurturing. So while young feet may be soft and sensitive, requiring lighter pressure than adult feet, don't delay introducing your children to reflexology early in life.

I have discovered over the years that children really give themselves to reflexology sessions, especially children who for a variety of reasons are not touched enough in their lives by family members, or who are mistreated physically. Hyperactive children calm down with reflexology and sluggish children are stimulated and energized.

Children naturally indulge in fantasies and games, so accompany reflexology sessions with visualizations and affirmations that will make the child an active participant in the "reflexology game" and facilitate healing. Let the child come up with spontaneous images, or suggest easy, positive ones of your own. For example, you can imagine a dark purple bruise fading away like a puddle evaporating in the sunshine. Or imagine swollen glands shrinking to normal size like an old balloon losing air. Affirmations can be put in the form of jingles or rhymes.

GOOD STEPS: FOR INTRODUCING YOUNG CHILDREN TO REFLEXOLOGY

Use relaxation techniques that your child finds enjoyable. Keep each session short, about 10 minutes. Be gentle but firm to avoid tickling the child. Keep a hand on each foot and let your fingers curl around the foot, pressing and squeezing gently to provide a sensation of security. Let the child fidget if he or she wants to; keep the session loose and playful. Make it a game. Remember that holding the solar plexus point in both feet will have a calming effect.

TALKING TO CHILDREN THROUGH THEIR FEET

As with adults, reflexology with children opens up pathways of communication between doer and receiver. A tradition of reflexology between parents and children can keep those pathways open during troubling times when a child needs to talk about worries and problems with siblings, schoolmates, teachers, or even the other parent. Children need healers and counselors in their lives. Too many parents neglect these all-important roles, leaving them to physicians, psychiatrists, and school counselors. Possibly parents don't feel competent or comfortable playing these roles, but as in many things, children never perceive the so-called incompetence. Reflexology can provide the setting in which the child—and you—learn that a parent can be healer, counselor, and friend, as well as parent.

In former times families spent a lot of time working and playing together, sitting in one big room, telling stories, and sharing their hopes and dreams with one another. Today television, two-career marriages, divorced or single parenthood, school activities, and after-school jobs all work at depriving the family of important time together. Kids want to open up and talk, but often there just isn't time. Or when there is, they can easily detect that mother or father is only half listening; they know the parent is preoccupied with other worries. Reflexology not only brings parents and children together, but by its very nature it focuses attention on each other in a warm, loving, and undistracted way.

As children get older and their hands and arms become strong enough, they will want to return the favor and do reflexology on parents. Encourage them to do so because it makes them feel needed and more grown up. It also introduces them to their own healing talents. What's more, mutual sessions equalize the power relationship between their generation and your own. Children need to have positive experiences of growing up and becoming equals with adults. Reflexology gives them that sense of competence and importance. It shows them that they can nurture tired parents and help relieve their tension. In the process, parents and children together create a new model for family life, one that dissolves the rigid definitions of what it means to be a parent or a child.

Use reflexology to talk to children about how they are doing at school. Many children suffer from learning disabilities of one type or another, and pinpointing the exact problem can be tricky. If the disability is due to physical problems, such as poor eyesight or hearing, or brain damage, work the zones for the head and bodily parts affected. If the problem is of a personal or psychological nature, reflexology can help to balance the child's energies, open up avenues of communication, and provide intimate times together when you can discuss what might be at the root of the problem. Sometimes poor academic performance is caused by fear of failure, abusive treatment by schoolmates, lack of self-confidence or recognition by teachers, simple inattention, or a host of other social and emotional hang-ups that can be worked out by talking them over with wise, comforting parents. As in all parent-child relationships, the bonding that occurs may provide the strength to help a child through difficult times at school; and that bonding itself can be strengthened by important rituals of health and relaxation such as reflexology.

Billy, the twelve-year-old son of a client of mine, was going through a moody, nontalkative period. His father, a warm and compassionate individual, was troubled over this. He convinced Billy to let him do reflexology on him. After a few sessions, the boy really "turned on to it" (as he put it), and began to open up and talk about his problems at school, the major one of which was his desire to try out for the softball team. A gawky, somewhat uncoordinated boy, he was afraid of failing and making a fool of himself. During reflexology sessions, he and his father talked about many things, and eventually the boy felt much better about himself, to the point that he eagerly tried out for the team and made second string. Interestingly, he also overcame a great deal of his uncoordination. Bill was so thrilled and so convinced that reflexology could work wonders that he asked his dad to continue the sessions all through the season. My client was happy for his son, naturally, but also amazed at how reflexology created a more open and trusting relationship between the two of them, especially during the teenage years when it is so natural for a child to pull away from a parent.

Remember: before each routine in this chapter, set up the environment as described in Chapter Three. Prepare the materials needed such as lotion, towel, and cornstarch. Create the appropriate mood with lighting and music. Review the person's health history. Check the feet for cuts, bruises, sores, corns, or calluses. If necessary, clean the feet with a warm washcloth or handiwipe. Clear and center yourself.

GOOD STEPS: FOR IMPROVING COMMUNICATION WITH CHILDREN

1.   Relax both feet with relaxation techniques, and end by holding the solar plexus point in both feet.

2.   As you work the points for a complete session, play a game called "Problems and Sole-utions." Ask your child at the end of the relaxation session to tell you one important problem that he is having at school, at home, with friends, or whatever. Then tell the child that while you are working on the right foot, you will be "working the problem out." As you begin to work the left foot, tell the child you are "working in healing ideas" that will flow through the child's thoughts and provide a solution to the problem. When you finish the left foot, the child tells you the solution he has come up with and how it will be enacted.

3.   Hold the solar plexus point in both feet, and end with breeze strokes.

GOOD STEPS: FOR TEACHING CHILDREN ABOUT THEIR BODIES

Use reflexology to teach children anatomy. As you move around on the foot, tell the child what area of the body each point that you are working refers to, and ask if she can indicate where on the body that part is. Soon the child will know where different parts of the body are, and where the corresponding points are on the foot. It will also get the child used to talking about her body and what the various parts are for.

FAMILY FOOT TIME

Reflexology among brothers and sisters is a wonderful way to ward off, or at least temper, sibling rivalry. It gives children a positive, constructive way to be together. Working each other's feet might be one of the few ways they show affection during the years when it isn't "cool" to admit they love each other—or touch each other.

GOOD STEPS: FOR ENCOURAGING WEEKLY REFLEXOLOGY IN THE FAMILY

Make a grid chart with the names of family members down the left and the days of the week across the top. At the beginning of the week all must indicate on the chart which day(s) they would like a reflexology session, and then sign their names in the boxes where they will have time to give a session.

BABY FEET

Even a newborn is not too young to receive reflexology. Of course, the child's foot might be no bigger than your thumb, so go easy. In fact, all that is needed in the first few months of life when a baby's bones are soft and rubbery is gentle rubbing and massaging. Most loving parents do this quite naturally. But as a reflexologist you will know that there is more going on than just oohs and aahs. You'll know gentle techniques for relaxing the foot and the whole baby. Get the baby used to having someone handle his feet in a loving yet systematic way. If a child is colicky or cries a lot for no apparent reason, apply gentle pressure to the solar plexus point. Often this is all that's needed to calm the little one down.

If you have big plans for your baby—and what parent doesn't?—include "foot plans." Prepare your child for a life of good health through reflexology. Take care of your children's feet right from the start. Don't tuck crib sheets in too tightly or cram children's feet into shoes and socks too early. In general, children should go barefoot until they are ready to walk. And let the child decide when it's time to walk. After all, there are a lot of steps ahead and children don't need to be forced into taking them before they are ready. When it's time, they will *want* to walk.

Unfortunately foot problems begin early. By age six, forty percent of American children have flat feet, toe deformities, or corns. So observe your children's feet carefully, getting them shoes that are the right size and shape for their activities. Up to age six, their shoes should be measured every four to six weeks to assure that their feet are not outgrowing them.

It's frustrating to watch little ones suffer pain, because we feel helpless and have no effective way to explain to them what's going wrong or to reassure them that they will feel better soon. Reflexology is one way to communicate with infants at these times in a physical, nonverbal manner, which on some level reassures the child that you are there and doing something good to make her feel better.

GOOD STEPS: FOR TEETHING

Each session should be only about 5 to 10 minutes. Give it when the baby is crying, or twice a day.

1. Relax both feet with relaxation techniques, and end by a thumb press on the solar plexus point in both feet. Relax each foot separately.

2. Thumb walk up the five zones of one foot and work the points suggested below.

3. Thumb walk up the five zones of the other foot and work the points suggested below.

4. Integrate relaxation techniques throughout the session as needed to help your baby relax when you encounter tender spots.

REFLEX AREA	TECHNIQUE	RATIONALE
NECK/CERVICALS	Thumb walk	• Improve circulation to gum and mouth area
LYMPH/NECK	Finger walk	• Fight infection
HEAD	Thumb and finger walk	• Improve circulation and energy in entire head region
GUMS AND MOUTH	Finger walk on the base of the toenails	• Encourage circulation and energy to gum and mouth area
ADRENALS	Rotate onto thumb	• Reduce inflammation

• Do relaxation techniques and thumb press on the solar plexus point in both feet, and end with breeze strokes.

GOOD STEPS: FOR SKIN IRRITATION

Each session should be only about 5 to 10 minutes, twice a day.

1.   Relax both feet with relaxation techniques, and end by a thumb press on the solar plexus point in both feet. Relax each foot separately.

2.   Thumb walk up the five zones of one foot and work the points suggested below.

3.   Thumb walk up the five zones of the other foot and work the points suggested below.

4.   Integrate relaxation techniques throughout the session as needed to help your child relax when you encounter tender spots.

REFLEX AREA	TECHNIQUE	RATIONALE
THYROID	Thumb walk	• Affect overall skin health
PITUITARY	Hook & back-up	• Control and regulate the functioning of all the glands
ENTIRE SPINE	Thumb walk	• Nervous and circulatory supply to entire body
DIAPHRAGM TO PELVIC LINE	Thumb walk on a diagonal	• Increase waste elimination
SPLEEN	Rotate onto thumb	• Release of substance that stimulates peristalsis
LIVER	Thumb walk on diagonal	• Help normalize production of bile • Blood cleansing
FROM BLADDER ON 45° ANGLE TO ZONE 3½	Thumb walk down	• Aid movement of waste material into rectal area
SIGMOID COLON	Hook & back-up	• Prevent or alleviate constipation

UP DESCENDING COLON TO WAISTLINE AND ACROSS ON TRANSVERSE COLON	Thumb walk	• Aid absorption of water and minerals • Aid elimination of waste
ILEOCECAL VALVE	Hook & back-up	• Regulate passage of food from small intestines to large intestines
UP ASCENDING COLON AND ACROSS TRANSVERSE COLON	Thumb walk	• Assist elimination of waste products and mucus
SMALL INTESTINES	Thumb walk on diagonal	• Improve peristaltic action for elimination of toxins and irritants
KIDNEYS	Rotate onto thumb	• Elimination of toxins • Filter system
ADRENALS	Rotate onto thumb	• Produce cortisone to reduce inflammation • Water balance

• Do relaxation techniques and thumb press on the solar plexus point in both feet, and end with breeze strokes.

Suggested Visualization:

If the child is old enough, let the child imagine he is in a very safe, clean, calm place playing comfortably with favorite toys while you or another loved one watch over him.

COMMON CHILDHOOD ILLNESSES

Common childhood illnesses will come and go, but reflexology should be a constant. Not only will it help kids get over their ailments more quickly, but we have found that children who get regular treatments come down less often with colds, upset stomachs, earaches, sore throats, even car sickness. Treat your child's body in a loving way, provide moments of deep relaxation and feeling good, and the child will have a stronger immune system. Kids will miss fewer school days as well as the activities they "really enjoy."

GOOD STEPS: FOR ALLEVIATING A FEVER

Do the following session about five minutes every half hour until the fever breaks.

1.   Relax both feet with relaxation techniques, and end by a thumb press on the solar plexus point in both feet. Relax each foot separately.

2.   Thumb walk up the five zones of one foot and work the points suggested below.

3.   Thumb walk up the five zones of the other foot and work the points suggested below.

4.   Integrate relaxation techniques throughout the session as needed to help your child relax when you encounter tender spots.

REFLEX AREA	TECHNIQUE	RATIONALE
THYROID AREA	Thumb walk	• Control metabolic rates which have a direct effect on heat production
LYMPH DRAINAGE IN NECK	Finger walk	• Lymph important in destroying bacteria
HYPOTHALAMUS	Hook & back-up	• Control body temperature
PITUITARY	Hook & back-up	• Control activity of all other glands
SPLEEN	Rotate onto thumb	• Defense mechanism—will fight off infection
LIVER	Thumb walk on a diagonal	• Help release toxins • Regulation of body heat
ADRENALS	Rotate onto thumb	• Fight inflammation • Maintain mineral balance
LYMPH AREA IN GROIN	Finger walk	• Drain viral infections from tissue spaces
PITUITARY	Hook & back-up	• Control activity of all other glands

•   Do relaxation techniques and thumb press on the solar plexus point in both feet, and end with breeze strokes.

Suggested Visualization:

Let the child imagine she is standing under a cool waterfall or playing under the sprinkler on the lawn on a hot summer day.

GOOD STEPS: FOR ALLEVIATING INFECTION

Each session should last 10 to 15 minutes, twice a day.

1.   Relax both feet with relaxation techniques, and end by a thumb press on the solar plexus point in both feet. Relax each foot separately.

2.   Thumb walk up the five zones of one foot and work the points suggested below.

3.   Thumb walk up the five zones of the other foot and work the points suggested below.

4.   Integrate relaxation techniques throughout the session as needed to help your child relax when you encounter tender spots.

REFLEX AREA	TECHNIQUE	RATIONALE
LYMPHATIC AREA OF CHEST BETWEEN FIRST AND SECOND TOES	Finger walk	• Lymphatic system absorbs waste products and toxins
TONSILS	Thumb walk and finger walk	• Stimulate tonsils, which are part of the body's defense system
PITUITARY	Hook & back-up	• Stimulate all endocrine glands
HEAD	Thumb walk down back of toes Finger walk down front of toes	• Stimulate circulation to head and neck area • Revitalize blood flow and energy to head and neck area
LYMPHATIC/GROIN	Finger walk	• Stimulate lymph areas in lower body
THYMUS	Thumb walk	• Help fight infection, especially in young children
SPLEEN	Rotate onto thumb	• Enhance production of antibodies to fight infection
POINTS ON FOOT THAT CORRESPOND TO INFECTED AREA	Stimulate	• Facilitate healing of the infected area
ADRENALS	Rotate and pivot onto thumb	• Help fight infection in body • Produce hormones which reduce inflammation • (The entire body is overworked during infection)

- Do relaxation techniques and thumb press on the solar plexus point in both feet, and end with breeze strokes.

Suggested Visualization:

Have the child imagine she is standing in a fresh breeze in the middle of a mountain meadow, playing with a favorite friend or family pet.

GOOD STEPS: FOR RESPIRATORY AILMENTS (ASTHMA, ALLERGIES, COLDS)

Each session should last 15 minutes, 2 or 3 times a week.

1. Relax both feet with relaxation techniques, and end by a thumb press on the solar plexus point in both feet. Relax each foot separately.

2. Thumb walk up the five zones of one foot and work the points suggested below.

3. Thumb walk up the five zones of the other foot and work the points suggested below.

4. Integrate relaxation techniques throughout the session as needed to help your child relax when you encounter tender spots.

REFLEX AREA	TECHNIQUE	RATIONALE
ENTIRE CHEST REGION	Thumb walk	• Break up congestion
LUNGS AND CHEST	Lung press	• Relax chest muscles
BRONCHIAL AREA	Thumb walk	• Relax smooth muscle of bronchials
DIAPHRAGM	Rotate onto thumb	• Facilitate deep breathing
LYMPH DRAINAGE/ CHEST	Finger walk	• Help break up congestion

THYMUS	Thumb walk	• Stimulate energy & strengthen immune system
RIDGE OF SHOULDER AND NECK LINE	Thumb walk and finger walk	• Help to free energy and blood flow from shoulders and neck to head, eyes, ears, nose
ALL TOES, ESPECIALLY MIDDLE THIRD OF EACH TOE	Thumb walk	• Open sinus cavities and nasal passageways
THROAT, TONSILS	Finger walk front and back base of toes	• All reflex areas to head go from back to front of toes
PITUITARY	Hook & back-up	• Control hormonal release to help all endocrine glands operate at a more optimal level
SPLEEN	Rotate onto thumb	• Balance immune function
ILEOCECAL VALVE	Hook & back-up	• Help regulate mucus levels in body
ADRENALS	Rotate onto thumb (work frequently during session)	• Help produce hormones that are anti-inflammitants • Adrenaline relaxes large airways in lungs
OVARIES AND TESTICLES	Small circular finger rotations	• Reproductive organs produce hormones used by the adrenal glands which can help the body cope with allergies
UTERUS AND PROSTATE	Rotate onto finger	• Same as for ovaries and testicles
LYMPH AND GROIN	Finger walk	• Balance immune function

• Do relaxation techniques and thumb press on the solar plexus point in both feet, and end with breeze strokes.

Suggested Visualization:

Have the child imagine himself healthy and happy playing alone in a huge room full of his favorite toys.

SICK IN BED

Being confined indoors or in bed can be boring, even for kids who enjoy staying at home cuddled up in the winter. Eventually even they get tired of being sick. Bed rest is always recommended for speedy recovery, but sometimes it's hard to keep restless, active kids in bed. Reflexology sessions can break up the long days of inactivity and give them something fun to look forward to. In addition, it stimulates the nervous system and improves circulation, which can grow sluggish without normal exercise. We also find that childhood illnesses, as well as simple colds and flu, don't linger if the patient receives reflexology in addition to traditional medical remedies.

Raising a chronically ill or disabled child can require heroic commitment from every member of the family. Family life will not be normal. Parents are sure to suffer disappointment and maybe even guilt, thinking that somehow they are to blame; other children may grow resentful of the ill child who demands more attention or puts a damper on family activities. Loving and caring for a disabled child can generate enormous amounts of stress. Reflexology can come to the rescue, especially for the ill or disabled child. It can alleviate boredom, improve circulation, and even become a kind of social activity if you teach the child's friends to do reflexology. Visits from peers can be more than just chitchat and games of gin rummy. The children can visit with a higher purpose of being part of the health care team.

On many levels the family with a disabled child needs relief and relaxation, time for meditation and reflection. Reflexology is not a panacea, but it can provide the quiet time of being together, releasing physical tension in the body, and renewing your commitment to providing the best family life you can.

Fear often accompanies illness, especially lingering illnesses—fear on the part of the child that she will never get well, perhaps even die; fear on the part of adults that they will not treat the illness correctly. Fear is usually irrational and may lead the child to actually fight off proper care by not eating or drinking fluids, refusing medications, kicking off blankets, or not staying in bed. Reflexology can act as a gentle reassurance that everything will be all right. It can alleviate parents' fear also, because having reflexology at their disposal lessens their feeling of powerlessness in dealing with their child's illness.

David, the teenage son of one of my associates, was a hyperactive child and burned off a lot of energy working for a bicycle messenger service. One day he was hit by a car and injured his knee. It required surgery and David was laid up for several months. My associate organized the boy's friends and neighbors, as well as other family members, to come over and give him reflexology sessions even while he was confined to bed with his leg in a cast. The sessions gave David a measure of social life and even contributed to his recovery, allowing him to reduce the amount of pain medication.

GOOD STEPS: FOR SOMEONE CONFINED TO BED

Each session should last 20 minutes, twice a day.

1. Relax both feet with relaxation techniques, and end by a thumb press on the solar plexus point in both feet. Relax each foot separately.

2. Thumb walk up the five zones of one foot and work the points suggested below.

3. Thumb walk up the five zones of the other foot and work the points suggested below.

4. Integrate relaxation techniques throughout the session as needed to help your partner relax when you encounter tender spots.

REFLEX AREA	TECHNIQUE	RATIONALE
CHEST/LUNGS	Thumb walk	• Encourage deep breathing • Prevent lung infections/pneumonia
HEART	Thumb walk up zones	• Maintain positive circulation • Prevent blood clots
SOLAR PLEXUS	Thumb press	• Encourage deep inspiration
LYMPH DRAINAGE/ NECK, CHEST	Finger walk	• Remove fluids, toxins and bacteria which accumulate during prolonged bed rest
THYROID	Thumb walk	• Affects metabolic rate
PITUITARY	Hook & back-up	• Stimulates activity of all major glands
SPINE	Thumb walk up, down, and across	• Improve circulation to entire body
SPLEEN	Rotate onto thumb	• Part of body's defense • Fights infection, through production of antibodies
ADRENALS	Rotate onto thumb	• Release cortisone • Fight inflammation • Produce adrenaline, which increases energy levels • Maintain more normal muscle tone
LYMPH/GROIN	Finger walk	• Stimulate lymphatic drainage of lower body
ENTIRE FOOT	Karate chops, punch and slap	• Stimulate entire body

• Do relaxation techniques and thumb press on the solar plexus point in both feet, and end with breeze strokes.

Suggested Visualization:

Have the child imagine he is floating on his back in a swimming pool or at the beach, with the sun pouring over his face and a refreshing breeze tickling his toes, without a care in the world.

BEDTIME RITUALS

Bedwetting is one of the banes of childhood. Many children seem to go through periods of it at one time or another. Pediatricians and psychologists have various remedies for it, some of which may work with some children and not with others. It is a perplexing problem, embarrassing for the child and other siblings and aggravating for parents. Most experts agree that the problem is usually emotional or psychological rather than physical, although sometimes practical physical strategies like having the child not drink water in the evening, having her urinate immediately before going to bed, or waking the child up halfway through the night for a trip to the bathroom may prevent the wet sheets in the morning. Nevertheless, the emotional causes rooted in stress and worry can remain.

Reflexology before bedtime (and regularly during the week) will relax and balance the child, helping her to cope with the deeper worries and tensions. Also, try reflexology if your child suffers from insomnia. Often children are tired enough after a busy day to sleep soundly, but worries and anxieties can prevent them from nodding off, just as with adults. A session before bedtime often assures a good night's sleep.

A friend of mine was a counselor a few years ago at a summer camp. He likes to tell about a camper named Spike, one of the "toughs" who bullied smaller campers. He was tough, all right—except at bedtime. The first three nights he wet his bed! Embarrassed by the wet sheets in the morning, Spike would torment other kids all the more to compensate. My friend checked with the boy's parents and learned that he hadn't wet his bed in years, so he was probably just reacting to his own fears of being away from home. The counselor decided to use a little tenderness on this tough guy. On the fourth night, he talked Spike into letting him do some reflexology on him right after lights-out. Whatever fears were troubling the boy seemed to abate, and Spike never wet his bed again. He also became less of a bully, and by the end of the camping season had a reasonably friendly relationship with his cabin mates.

GOOD STEPS: FOR GETTING READY FOR BED (ESPECIALLY FOR BEDWETTERS)

Each session should last 15 minutes at bedtime.

1.   Relax both feet with relaxation techniques, and end by a thumb press on the solar plexus point in both feet. Relax each foot separately.

2.   Thumb walk up the five zones of one foot and work the points suggested below.

3.   Thumb walk up the five zones of the other foot and work the points suggested below.

4.   Integrate relaxation techniques throughout the session as needed to help your partner relax when you encounter tender spots.

REFLEX AREA	TECHNIQUE	RATIONALE
CHEST REGION	Thumb walk	• Open up chest to deepen breathing
DIAPHRAGM	Thumb walk	• Relax tension built up in chest region
SPINE	Thumb walk up, down, across, and rotate onto thumb	• Release tension • Balance nervous system, allowing for deep relaxation
SPINE	Spinal twist	• Relax spine and back muscles • Soothe nervous response
NECK	Thumb walk across and finger walk around	• Release tension in neck area
BRAIN	Roll	• Relax central nervous system
PITUITARY	Hook & back-up	• Release of hormones to regulate body activities

URETER	Thumb walk	• Aid water elimination
BLADDER, KIDNEYS	Rotate onto thumb	• Purify bloodstream
ADRENALS	Rotate onto thumb	• Balance energy

•   Do relaxation techniques and thumb press on the solar plexus point in both feet, and end with breeze strokes.

Suggested game: As you work the two big toes, have your child set two goals, one on each toe, of something he is looking forward to doing or having happen the next day.

Suggested Visualization:

Have the child imagine he is sleeping secure and safe at home, with his parents sleeping contentedly nearby in their own room. If the child likes, he can also imagine the family home surrounded with a big, glowing white parachute that keeps all the love inside and filters anything troubling out and away. Or, let the child simply imagine that his bed is surrounded by a big, glowing white parachute that keeps all harm away.

ENERGY: TOO MUCH, TOO LITTLE

Some children are hyperactive, others are sluggish. Of course, that's true of adults too; it's just that we don't make a big deal of it! We expect some people to be go-getters and others laid-back. But with children we rightly become concerned if the child seems too lethargic or too high-strung. Both conditions can prevent them from making the best use of the childhood years and may set patterns for later problems in development and adjustment. Both hyperactivity and sluggishness respond well to reflexology.

GOOD STEPS: FOR HYPERACTIVITY OR SLUGGISHNESS

Both these problems relate to the same areas of the body, so one routine will cover both.

Each session should last 10 to 15 minutes and be done 2 or 3 times a week.

1.   Relax both feet with relaxation techniques, and end by a thumb press on the solar plexus point in both feet. Relax each foot separately.

2.   Thumb walk up the five zones of one foot and work the points suggested below.

3.   Thumb walk up the five zones of the other foot, and work the points suggested below.

4.   Integrate relaxation techniques throughout the session as needed to help your child relax when you encounter tender spots.

REFLEX AREA	TECHNIQUE	RATIONALE
DIAPHRAGM	Thumb walk across and rotate onto thumb	• Induce breathing more freely to relax and energize
THYMUS	Thumb walk	• Stimulate energy
THYROID	Thumb walk	• Speed up or slow down bodily processes and activities
BRAIN	Roll & rock	• Balance central nervous system
PITUITARY	Hook & back-up	• Regulate activity of other glands
ACROSS PANCREAS ABOVE WAIST LINE (PRIMARILY ON LEFT FOOT)	Thumb walk	• Control over blood sugar levels in body • Direct effect on energy output
LIVER	Thumb walk across	• Flush toxins that could be creating sluggishness or irritability

| ADRENALS | Rotate onto thumb | • Produce adrenaline for balance of energy and control heart/lung activity |
| | | • Mineral balance |

• Do relaxation techniques and thumb press on the solar plexus point in both feet, and end with breeze strokes.

Suggested Visualization:

Let the child imagine she is playing her favorite game with her best friends in a beautiful, flower-filled wood.

BROKEN BONES AND BRUISES

Athletic injuries in children can take a double toll: first because of the physical injury itself, and second because of the inability of young children to understand the unfairness of it all. Granted, physical disability is a disappointment for athletes of any age, but it can be exceptionally devastating for children who haven't had the experience yet of learning to handle setbacks and bad luck. Young people dream big, and dreams that don't come true leave big holes in their lives. At times like this it's important for parents to be on hand to ease their children's pain and get them through periods of feeling worthless. Reflexology can temper the moodiness or hostility that extreme disappointment can produce. Regular sessions will give the disappointed athlete something positive to do to shorten recovery time. You might even schedule them during the hours after school when the rest of the team is practicing, since this would be the time when the child would probably feel most left out and helpless.

GOOD STEPS: FOR ATHLETES

See Chapter Ten.

TEENAGE TURMOIL: ACNE

Families go through a lot of turmoil during the teenage years. In parents it can produce ulcers, in teens acne (although it's not uncommon these days to find ulcers in adolescents and acne in adults). There are several physical causes of acne, such as hormonal changes, body chemistry, diet, hygiene, and hereditary tendencies; and yet it seems that flare-ups are often directly related to stressful situations that rev up the oil glands. Like Murphy's law, acne breaks out at the worst possible times—before important dates, on the first day of class, right before the yearbook pictures are taken. Emotional upheaval, worry, tension—and in the teenage years these can occur hourly—all take their toll on the face. Reflexology is not a substitute for good hygiene, eating sensibly, and using the right medications, but it can certainly relieve the effects of stress, balance the body chemistry, and keep adolescents on a more stable emotional keel.

TEENAGE TURMOIL: DRUGS AND ALCOHOL

Many teens experiment with alcohol and drugs; some abuse them; a few become addicts and alcoholics. The problem is complicated and challenging even for the professionals who specialize in teenage addictions. There are no easy solutions. Professional reflexologists have joined the care teams that are treating teenage alcoholics and drug abusers, and the results are impressive. As in any recovery program, a methodology works best on people who can handle stress, relax, and let the natural healing properties of their own bodies go to work. Reflexology is proving to be a great method for helping addicted teenagers bring their lives back into balance.

The natural moodiness of adolescents is never easy to live with, and it can be devastating to family life when drugs or alcohol escalate their moodiness into abusiveness, irresponsibility, and physical violence. If your own children are having problems at home or school that could lure them into escaping through drugs and drink, try reflexology before the minor troubles escalate into serious emotional and behavioral problems with school authorities or the law. If you suspect a child is abusing drugs or alcohol, seek outside professional help such as Alateen or a responsible drug therapy program. School counselors or family physicians can advise you on this.

GOOD STEPS: FOR DRUG AND ALCOHOL ABUSE

See Chapter Eleven.

TEENAGE TURMOIL: SEX

Teenage sexuality can create all kinds of troubles and worries for the teens themselves as well as their parents. It is a complex and difficult issue for everyone: what to say, what to do, what not to say and not to do—for both parents and kids. I like to think that with many teenagers reflexology could alleviate some of the reasons they engage in sex before they are really prepared for it. Some teens leap into sexual adventures simply because they want to be touched and comforted in a physical way. Reflexology in the family, as well as with boyfriends and girlfriends, can be an alternate for sexual activity until a teen is physically and emotionally ready. Reflexology and some forms of massage can help adolescents explore and appreciate their bodies without the complications of social and sexual roles. Even in romantic relationships, some young couples may find that these ways of being tender and affectionate with each other are actually preferable to heavy sexual involvement.

Some teenage girls who become pregnant are choosing to have and keep their babies even though it may wreck their social lives, endanger their health, curtail their education, and be a financial burden on them and their own parents. Why? One answer is that they see in the love of a newborn baby the love and affection they do not get elsewhere, either from their parents or from their peers. They put all their hopes in the new baby and themselves as new mothers. Many of them are sadly disappointed. Reflexology from parents could be an acknowledgment of love and appreciation; it could strengthen the bonds that will keep teens looking toward the family for love and acceptance. It might also tip the scales in favor of their waiting until a more appropriate time to begin a family.

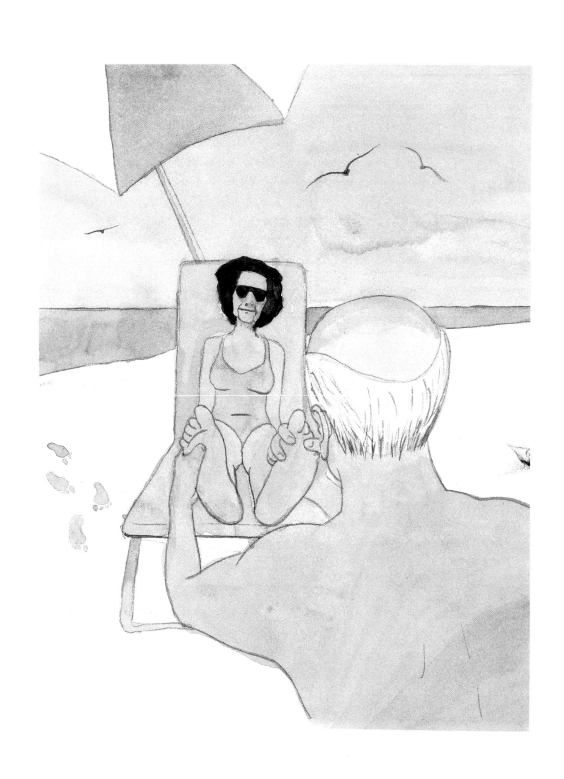

CHAPTER NINE

AFTER WALKING MANY MILES:

REFLEXOLOGY IN THE GOLDEN YEARS

The older generation has walked many miles and should be able to enjoy their Golden Years as wise and patient counselors to the younger generations following after them. They ought to be regarded as vital, supportive members of the family; and yet they often end up being treated as the weakest links in the family chain, requiring the support and help of others. What has gone wrong?

As we age, the immune system deteriorates and makes us more susceptible to disease. Eighty-five percent of those over sixty-five have at least three chronic ailments. They also lack energy and get tired more easily. Fatigue or lack of energy, coupled with a poor diet that can be due either to lack of interest, less money, or loneliness, can zap one's enthusiasm for life and create a kind of boredom and indifference to the family as well as the world in general.

Consequently we begin to look upon the older generation in a strange light. We start to think of aging as a disease in itself, even though it is a natural process. Disease, strictly speaking, is a disruption of the life process, a condition that interrupts the natural bodily functions. Aging, on the other hand, is part of nature's plan, and even though part of the plan is that the body slows down and becomes weaker, it is not an indication that anything is wrong. After all, a young person's body slows down and grows weaker after a hard day or a busy weekend, and we think nothing is unusual. We accept that there are different rhythms and energies at different times in our lives. And yet, when it comes to senior citizens, we look upon these changing rhythms as disease. It is a sad commentary on our obsession with youth and beauty that we often even stop touching older people simply because they look and feel "different."

Reflexology is a natural for senior citizens. It can help them feel better, relieve many aches and pains, provide a way for older couples to continue physical intimacy with each other, and offer them a useful role in the family and neighborhood. It is a natural because health is a major concern among the older generations. The "retirement syndrome" in our society has concentrated large numbers of retired people together in communities where chronic ailments, operations, hospitalizations, and deaths become the major topic of conversation. In fact, with many older persons health (or illness) is an obsession. A depressing self-fulfilling cycle emerges in which undue worry over minor aches produces stress that weakens the immune system further, causing older people to be even more susceptible to illnesses. This in turn generates even more worry, sleepless nights, and incessant gossip among friends, and the net result is to escalate the concern and worry over disease.

What can older persons do? They can become a vital force to break up this vicious cycle. They can become healers who can bring new energy and rejuvenation to themselves and their own mates as well as to other senior citizens in their communities. In fact, practicing reflexology on themselves and others will strengthen their roles in the family as parents and grandparents. They will overcome their sense of helplessness and assuage the fears of aging. Part of the wisdom of old age should be the knowledge of and remedies for staying healthy.

Older persons can do reflexology on themselves as long as they can still cross one leg over the other. Even if stiff joints prevent this, reflexology can become part of the bath ritual where the sides of the tub provide support for reaching the feet. This is an excellent time to do reflexology no matter what age you are. I usually do some work on my own feet every time I take a bath.

Remember: before each routine in this chapter, set up the environment as described in Chapter Three. Prepare the materials needed such as lotion, towel, and cornstarch. Create the appropriate mood with lighting and music. Review the person's health history. Check the feet for cuts, bruises, sores, corns, or calluses. If necessary, clean the feet with a warm washcloth or handiwipe. Clear and center yourself.

GOOD STEPS: FOR WORKING ON OLDER PEOPLE

There are several pointers to keep in mind when working on older feet:

- Often the toes tend to be more permanently bent and should not be unduly straightened out when doing reflexology. Work within the natural configuration of the toes. Gradually, they will loosen up and you'll be able to stretch and extend them more fully.

- Be careful to work lightly on areas of the skin with broken blood vessels. The small vessels in the feet tend to break with age and these areas need gentle treatment.

- When stretching out the leg at the beginning of a session, guard against applying too much force, especially if the person has had hip difficulties. Older hip joints can be brittle and not as flexible as younger ones.

- At any age you may hear crackling when rotating toes or feet. It may be even more noticeable with older people. This in itself doesn't mean that anything is wrong with the feet or that your technique is too rough. It is natural for bones and joints in the feet to crack and pop.

- Work seniors for shorter time periods, more frequently, and with a lighter touch.

COMMON AILMENTS OF THE MATURE YEARS

Some of the more common ailments typical of the mature years are discussed in the following sections. All of them respond well to reflexology.

Arthritis

Inflammation in the joints can be reduced by the natural production of cortisone from the adrenals. Often, older people take cortisone supplements to relieve the burning pain. Serious problems and side effects can result, including the adrenals' shutting down their own production. Professional reflexologists have noticed that with regular reflexology sessions that stimulate the adrenals, arthritis sufferers can sometimes reduce or eliminate their dependence on pharmaceutical cortisone (only with their physicians' approval, of course).

In addition to the adrenals, work the specific points that correspond to the affected body area. Also, people with arthritis in their hands should be encouraged to do reflexology because the exercise it gives their fingers and wrists can prevent flare-ups.

GOOD STEPS: FOR ARTHRITIS

Each session should last 15 to 20 minutes and be done once a day.

1. Relax both feet with relaxation techniques, and end by a thumb press on the solar plexus point in both feet. Relax each foot separately.

2. Thumb walk up the five zones of one foot and work the points suggested below.

3. Thumb walk up the five zones of the other foot and work the points suggested below.

4. Integrate relaxation techniques throughout the session as needed to help your partner relax when you encounter tender spots.

REFLEX AREA	TECHNIQUE	RATIONALE
DIAPHRAGM	Rotate onto thumb	• Release muscular tension
ARM, SHOULDER, ELBOW AND WRIST AREAS	Thumb and finger walk	• Facilitate healing • Improve circulation and nerve impulses
HIP, KNEE, LEG, AND ANKLE AREAS	Finger walk	• Facilitate healing
SPINE	Thumb walk up, down, and across	• Increase flexibility • Normalize nervous responses
SOLAR PLEXUS	Return to often, apply gentle pressure	• Relax breathing
PARATHYROIDS	Thumb walk	• Balance calcium and potassium levels
LIVER	Thumb walk	• Filter toxins
KIDNEYS	Thumb walk and rotate onto thumb	• Reduce edema and release water that can accumulate in joints • Filters out toxins and irritants through urinary excretion
ADRENALS	Thumb walk and rotate onto thumb	• Mineral balance • Improve muscle tone • Reduce inflammation with cortisone production, which eases inflammation
REFERRAL AREAS FOR AFFECTED AREA	Thumb and finger walk	• Clear energy throughout the zone
ENTIRE FOOT	Side-to-side wringing	• Relax tension that brings on and aggravates arthritis

- Do relaxation techniques and thumb press on the solar plexus point in both feet, and end with breeze strokes.

Suggested Visualization:

Let your partner see and feel himself floating in a pool of healing, green water that is easing all the pain and stiffness away.

Diabetes

Reflexology produces good results with adult-onset diabetes, especially if the sessions begin shortly after it is diagnosed. (Adults who were juvenile diabetics do not respond as quickly to reflexology because the disease is well established in their bodies.) One client of mine discovered after regular reflexology sessions that the triglyceride level in her blood dropped sufficiently enough that her doctor discontinued her prescriptions of insulin.

A former student in his mid-sixties named Stewart had an older friend who was dying of cancer. The friend was also diabetic. Stewart gave him short reflexology sessions several times a week, primarily as a way to spend time with him and also in the hopes that relaxation would help the older man in his final days. Stewart focused on the pancreas area because of the man's diabetes. At one point, the man decided, on his own and without telling anyone, to stop taking his insulin dosage because he was growing more discouraged and didn't want to prolong his life. Yet a remarkable thing happened. When the doctors discovered what the man had done, they checked his blood sugar level and were amazed that it had remained the same as when he was on the medication! The only way way they could account for it was Stewart's reflexology work, which stimulated the pancreas to regulate its own insulin production.

GOOD STEPS: FOR DIABETES

Each session should last 15 to 20 minutes and be done 3 times a week.

1.   Relax both feet with relaxation techniques, and end by a thumb press on the solar plexus point in both feet. Relax each foot separately.

2. Thumb walk up the five zones of one foot and work the points suggested below.

3. Thumb walk up the five zones of the other foot and work the points suggested below.

4. Integrate relaxation techniques throughout the session as needed to help your partner relax when you encounter tender spots.

REFLEX AREA	TECHNIQUE	RATIONALE
HEART	Thumb walk	• Aid circulation
THYROID	Thumb walk	• Regulate metabolism
EYE AREA	Thumb walk	• Improve circulation
PITUITARY	Hook & back-up	• Balance endocrine function
SPINE	Thumb walk	• Stimulate nerve impulses to all parts of the body
LEG AND REFERRAL AREAS	Thumb walk	• Improve circulation
PANCREAS	Thumb walk across	• Encourage balance of hormones • Balance blood sugar levels
LIVER	Thumb walk across and on diagonal and rotate onto thumb	• Detoxify blood and improve fat digestion • Store and release glycogen, a form of sugar
INTESTINES	Thumb walk & pivot	• Promote optimum absorbtion of vitamins and minerals • Facilitate rapid excretion of waste • Altered blood glucose levels can cause diarrhea/constipation
KIDNEYS	Thumb walk and rotate onto thumb	• Encourage balanced elimination of fluids • Filter urine and excrete excess sugar
ADRENALS	Rotate onto thumb	• Balance energy levels • Secrete hormones involved with protein and carbohydrate metabolism

- Do relaxation techniques and thumb press on the solar plexus point in both feet, and end with breeze strokes.

Suggested Visualization:

Let your partner imagine herself healthy, strong, and happy, and surrounded by everything and everyone she has ever wanted in her life.

Vision and Hearing

An elderly man whom I treated recently was dismayed because as he got older he had to curtail the number of hours he could read each day. Reading had been one of his favorite pastimes throughout his life and gave him a lot of pleasure in his mature years especially because it kept him abreast of the times and mentally alert. He hated to give it up, but when he came to me he was only able to read about a half hour a day. After several reflexology sessions, he could extend his daily reading to two hours.

GOOD STEPS: FOR VISION AND HEARING LOSS

Each session should last 15 minutes and be done every day.

1.   Relax both feet with relaxation techniques, and end by a thumb press on the solar plexus point in both feet. Relax each foot separately.

2.   Thumb walk up the five zones of one foot and work the points suggested below.

3.   Thumb walk up the five zones of the other foot and work the points suggested below.

4.   Integrate relaxation techniques throughout the session as needed to help your partner relax when you encounter tender spots.

REFLEX AREA	TECHNIQUE	RATIONALE
ARMS AND SHOULDERS	Thumb walk	• Relaxation
SPINE	Thumb walk up, down, and across	• Stimulate nervous system
SPINE	Spinal twist	• Stretch spine
SPINE	Rotate onto thumb	• Loosen spine and improve circulation
NECK AND CERVICALS	Thumb walk and finger walk around	• Enhance relaxation in neck muscles, thus enhancing blood and nerve impulses to face and brain
NECK	Toe rotation/hang on ridge	• Relax and loosen neck muscles
SINUS, EYES, AND EARS REGION	Thumb walk down and across	• Reduce pressure • Open passageways • Eliminate blockages
PITUITARY	Hook & back-up	• Regulate hormonal secretions in endocrine glands
NECK AND HEAD	Toe boogie	• Relax and loosen neck and head muscles
BRAIN	Roll and rock	• Stimulate optic nerve • Stimulate sensory receptors
LIVER	Thumb walk	• Neutralize toxins in the blood and combat bacterial infection
KIDNEYS	Rotate onto thumb	• Cleanse and purify blood • Clear energy in same zone as eye and inner ear
ADRENALS	Rotate onto thumb	• Secrete hormones which fight infection and balance minerals

•   Do relaxation techniques and thumb press on the solar plexus point in both feet, and end with breeze strokes.

Suggested Visualization:

Let your partner imagine he is seeing his favorite sights in brilliant color and focus; or hearing his favorite sounds with all their nuance, and clarity.

Stomach Problems

Older people often suffer from various stomach disorders, most of them resulting in indigestion or heartburn. After my own grandmother had most of her stomach removed, she discovered that she could not keep her meals down. At one point it became a very serious problem because she risked undernourishment. Like so many of her generation, she had a lot of time on her hands and would tend to sit around and worry about it. Worry led to tension that only compounded the problem at every meal. I worked on her every day so that she relaxed enough to be able to keep at least one meal down. Her problem and other stomach ailments responded very well to reflexology.

GOOD STEPS: FOR INDIGESTION

Each session should last 15 minutes before heavy meals.

1.   Relax both feet with relaxation techniques, and end by a thumb press on the solar plexus point in both feet. Relax each foot separately.

2.   Thumb walk up the five zones of one foot and work the points suggested below.

3.   Thumb walk up the five zones of the other foot and work the points suggested below.

4.   Integrate relaxation techniques throughout the session as needed to help your partner relax when you encounter tender spots.

REFLEX AREA	TECHNIQUE	RATIONALE
CHEST	Thumb walk	• Deepen breathing
NECK	Toe rotation	• Relax neck muscles
THROAT AND ESOPHAGUS	Thumb walk	• Relax smooth muscles
MOUTH AREA	Finger walk	• Encourage digestive enzyme production and release • Strengthen gums and teeth
SPINE (THORACIC AND LUMBAR)	Thumb walk and rotate onto thumb	• Stimulate spinal nerves to aid digestion
SIGMOID COLON	Thumb walk along	• Relax the area and allow free movement of waste products
DESCENDING COLON TRANSVERSE COLON	Thumb walk up Thumb walk across	• Encourage absorbtion of nutrients and water • Promote regular peristaltic movement of waste
STOMACH	Thumb walk across	• Release gastric juices • Aid stomach movement
PANCREAS	Thumb walk across	• Promote release of digestive enzymes • Move food along intestinal tract • Aid digestion
LIVER	Thumb walk and rotate onto thumb	• Stimulate production of bile • Detoxification of blood
GALLBLADDER	Rotate onto thumb	• Encourage proper bile release
ILEOCECAL VALVE	Hook & back-up	• Encourage absorption of nutrients and water
ASCENDING COLON	Thumb walk up	• Promote regular peristaltic movement of waste
SMALL INTESTINES AND DUODENUM	Thumb walk diagonally across	• Encourage release of digestive enzymes • Improve intestinal movement • Break down food and move it through intestinal tract

- Do relaxation techniques and thumb press on the solar plexus point in both feet, and end with breeze strokes.

Suggested Visualization:

Let your partner imagine she is lying under a beautiful blue gauzy canopy, and that a beautiful, pulsating blue and gold light is soothing pain and discomfort away.

Constipation and Other Elimination Problems

Older people are prone to suffer constipation, which can be caused by tension, poor diet, indigestion, and inactivity. Working the liver, gallbladder, and colon reflex areas can prevent constipation. Lower-back problems, often caused by excessive sitting, also have impact on the colon and the elimination process.

Prostate problems in men seem to have been ready made for reflexology! Most reflexologists will attest to a high success rate with this ailment. Regular sessions break up the congestion in the prostate gland and allow urination to function more naturally.

A woman client of mine who suffered from bladder problems was feeling left out of her family because when the rest of them went off on weekend picnics and short trips she felt like a nuisance having to stop so often to urinate. Eventually she declined to go with them even though she hated to stay home alone and miss out on the fun. Reflexology helped her bladder get back on a more normal schedule so that she could travel with the family and not have to ask for bathroom stops.

GOOD STEPS: FOR CONSTIPATION AND DIARRHEA

Each session should last 20 to 30 minutes and be done once a day.

1. Relax both feet with relaxation techniques, and end by a thumb press on the solar plexus point in both feet. Relax each foot separately.

2. Thumb walk up the five zones of one foot and work the points suggested below.

3.   Thumb walk up the five zones of the other foot and work the points suggested below.

4.   Integrate relaxation techniques throughout the session as needed to help your partner relax when you encounter tender spots.

REFLEX AREA	TECHNIQUE	RATIONALE
HEART	Thumb walk up and across	• Better circulation and gas exchange
DIAPHRAGM LINE	Rotate onto thumb	• Stimulate regular breathing patterns and relaxation
LUNGS AND CHEST	Lung press	• Relax chest region • Deepen breathing
THROAT, ESOPHAGUS, THYROID AND PARATHYROIDS	Thumb walk all around	• Aid the movement of food into the stomach • Normalize metabolic rate • Regulate minerals involved with muscle contractions (peristalsis)
MOUTH AREA	Finger walk	• Encourage production and release of digestive enzymes
NECK	Toe rotation	• Relax and loosen neck muscles for general relaxation
PITUITARY, PINEAL AND HYPOTHALAMUS	Hook & back-up	• Stimulate glandular functions to balance emotional stress
SPINE (EMPHASIS ON LOWER SPINE)	Thumb walk up, down and across	• Stimulate nerves which feed into colon and bladder
SPINE	Spinal twist	• Relax chest region and ease breathing
STOMACH	Thumb walk	• Encourage muscular activity • Encourage production of gastric juices and peristalsis

PANCREAS	Thumb walk across	• Stimulate production and release of pancreatic enzymes that aid in breakdown of food
SPLEEN	Rotate onto thumb	• Release of substance that stimulates peristalsis
SIGMOID COLON	Thumb walk down from bladder on 45° angle to zone 3½ Hook & back-up	• Aid movement of waste material into rectal area
UP DESCENDING COLON TO WAIST LINE AND ACROSS ON TRANSVERSE COLON	Thumb walk	• Aid absorption of water and minerals • Aid elimination of waste
SMALL INTESTINES BETWEEN WAIST LINE AND PELVIC LINE (BOTH FEET)	Thumb walk on a diagonal	• Improve absorption of nutrients from small intestines • Improve peristaltic action
KIDNEY	Rotate onto thumb	• Aid elimination of waste and water balance
LIVER	Thumb walk & rotate onto thumb	• Detoxify blood • Secrete bile • Many metabolic functions (fat, protein, etc.)
GALLBLADDER	Rotate onto thumb	• Encourage bile release, which assists in fat digestion
ADRENALS	Rotate onto thumb	• Control muscle tone • Produce hormones involved with water balance in the body
ILEOCECAL VALVE	Hook & back up	• Regulate passage of food from small intestines to large intestines
UP ASCENDING COLON AND ACROSS TRANSVERSE COLON	Thumb walk	• Assist elimination of waste products and mucus
CHRONIC AREA	Finger walk	• Improve muscle tone, circulation, etc. of pelvic organs

- Do relaxation techniques and thumb press on the solar plexus point in both feet, and end with breeze strokes.

Suggested Visualization:

Same as visualization for indigestion.

GOOD STEPS: FOR BLADDER PROBLEMS

Each session should last 20 to 30 minutes and be done once a day.

1. Relax both feet with relaxation techniques, and end by a thumb press on the solar plexus point in both feet. Relax each foot separately.

2. Thumb walk up the five zones of one foot and work the points suggested below.

3. Thumb walk up the five zones of the other foot and work the points suggested below.

4. Integrate relaxation techniques throughout the session as needed to help your partner relax when you encounter tender spots.

REFLEX AREA	TECHNIQUE	RATIONALE
DIAPHRAGM LINE	Rotate onto thumb	• Stimulate regular breathing patterns and relaxation
LUNGS AND CHEST	Lung press	• Relax chest region • Deepen breathing
HEART	Thumb walk up and across	• Better circulation and gas exchange

PITUITARY, PINEAL, AND HYPOTHALAMUS	Hook & back-up	• Stimulate glandular functions to regain emotional balance under stress
SPINE	Spinal twist	• Relax chest region and ease breathing
SPINE	Thumb walk up, down, and across	• Stimulate nerves which feed into colon and bladder
LIVER	Thumb walk & rotate onto thumb	• Detoxify blood • Secrete bile • Many metabolic functions (fat, protein, etc.)
BLADDER AND KIDNEYS	Thumb walk and rotate onto thumb	• Eliminate urine
ADRENALS	Rotate onto thumb	• Control muscle tone • Produce hormones involved with water balance in the body
PROSTATE	Rotate onto finger	• Release congestion • Help pressure off urethra if it is enlarged

•   Do relaxation techniques and thumb press on the solar plexus point in both feet, and end with breeze strokes.

Suggested Visualization:

Let your partner imagine his bladder surrounded with a whirling globe of cool, healing green, pink, or white light that is polishing and soothing away any pain or irritation. (The pain or irritation can be seen as another color that the protective globe is whirling away.)

Edema

Edema, the swelling of limbs and joints due to excess fluid retention, responds well to reflexology. Work gently on the feet if they are swollen, pushing the fluid up toward the leg during relaxation exercises. Also work the reflex points for any body parts that are swollen. Work referral areas if the feet are too painful to work.

GOOD STEPS: FOR EDEMA

Each session should last 15 to 20 minutes and be done 3 times a week. Elevate the feet or injured part.

1. Relax both feet with relaxation techniques, and end by a thumb press on the solar plexus point in both feet. Relax each foot separately.

2. Thumb walk up the five zones of one foot and work the points suggested below.

3. Thumb walk up the five zones of the other foot and work the points suggested below.

4. Integrate relaxation techniques throughout the session as needed to help your partner relax when you encounter tender spots.

REFLEX AREA	TECHNIQUE	RATIONALE
CHEST/LUNG/HEART	Thumb walk vertically	• Edema to extremities can be caused by congestion in heart/lung area or poor circulation to affected area
LYMPH DRAINAGE/ NECK, CHEST	Finger walk	• Release fluid in chest
PITUITARY GLAND	Hook & back-up	• Stimulate hormone release which affects other endocrine glands
SPINE	Thumb walk up, down, and across	• Increase neural integration
LIVER	Thumb walk diagonally across	• Part of portal circulation—congestion here can cause edema of legs • Detoxification functions
BLADDER, URETERS AND KIDNEYS	Thumb walk across and rotate onto thumb	• Balancing and eliminating water in the body

ADRENALS	Thumb walk and rotate onto thumb	• Balance minerals in the body • Produce hormones involved with fluid retention
LYMPH DRAIN	Finger walk	• Drain tissue spaces
PARTICULAR AREA THAT IS EDEMIC AND REFERRAL AREA	Thumb walk	• Relieve congestion

• Do relaxation techniques and thumb press on the solar plexus point in both feet, and end with breeze strokes.

Suggested Visualization:

Let your partner imagine a soft, gentle spring rain is moistening her body and washing away all cares and any extra water or heaviness through lavender rain pipes that run all the way down and through her body. Playing an environmental tape of a rainfall will really augment this effect! You can also ask your partner to imagine that tiny soft crystals are inside her body, polishing and loosening any extra water so it can run down the pipes and out into the world.

Cardiovascular Ailments

Heart attack, stroke, and high blood pressure are common ailments among older persons. Do reflexology as soon as possible after heart surgery, always checking with the doctor first. In emergencies, such as immediately after a heart attack or stroke, don't hesitate to grab a foot and begin working the heart reflexes and the pituitary after you have provided cardiopulmonary resuscitation (CPR) (or while someone else provides it), treated for shock, and called an ambulance. Family members often wonder what they can do while they wait for the ambulance. Well, if you know reflexology, you know what you should do.

As postoperative therapy, reflexology can help heart patients recover more quickly and get back to normal living. Many of my clients who have had open-heart surgery come to me with great difficulty walking and breathing. In less time than they and their doctors had expected, they are back to normal, dashing around town, going to luncheons, visiting friends, even playing sports.

GOOD STEPS: FOR HEART PROBLEMS

Each session should last 15 to 20 minutes and be done 2 or 3 times a week.

1.   Relax both feet with relaxation techniques, and end by a thumb press on the solar plexus point in both feet. Relax each foot separately.

2.   Thumb walk up the five zones of one foot and work the points suggested below.

3.   Thumb walk up the five zones of the other foot and work the points suggested below.

4.   Integrate relaxation techniques throughout the session as needed to help your partner relax when you encounter tender spots.

REFLEX AREA	TECHNIQUE	RATIONALE
LUNGS AND CHEST	Thumb walk in several directions	• Relaxation • Improve circulation and heart rate
LUNGS AND CHEST	Lung press	• Relax chest and deepen breathing • Facilitate better oxygenation of blood
HEART AREA	Thumb walk and rotate onto thumb	• Normalize heart rate
SHOULDER/ARM	Thumb walk	• Help circulation to heart

DIAPHRAGM LINE	Rotate onto thumb	• Release muscular tension in chest area
ADRENALS	Rotate onto thumb	• Release adrenaline, which stimulates heart contraction and dilates bronchials • Improve muscle tone
PITUITARY	Hook & back-up	• Stimulate the endocrine glands which influence heart rate, blood pressure, and respiration
BRAIN	Finger roll	• Plays a crucial part in how the heart functions
SPINE (PARTICULARLY THORACIC)	Thumb walk up, down, and across	• Regulate nerve impulses
SPINE	Spinal twist	• Stretch spine
SPINE	Spinal rotation	• Loosen spine and improve circulation
KIDNEYS	Thumb walk and rotate onto thumb	• Release water that places pressure on heart • Regulate mineral levels
COLON (ESPECIALLY SIGMOID)	Thumb walk on a diagonal	• Gas pockets create pressure on heart

• Do relaxation techniques and thumb press on the solar plexus point in both feet, and end with breeze strokes.

Suggested Visualization:

Let your partner imagine a pink-and-green-striped cabbage rose in the center of his chest (or, a pink rose with a green stem). Have the rose whirl around the heart area, and have your partner feel his entire chest fill up with joy. Let your partner imagine himself listening to a group of rosy-cheeked Christmas carolers, or encourage him to re-create an especially joyous and loving event from his own life.

Memory Loss

Everyone's memory begins to deteriorate in the adult years. In general, you won't be as sharp in your forties as you were in your thirties, and by the time you're in your golden years you may be distraught over the amount of factual information you can't remember. It's estimated that eighty-five percent of healthy people over sixty-five suffer some memory loss. Theories vary as to how and why we forget what we do, but we know that memory requires an interplay of natural chemicals produced in the brain as well as sufficient oxygen to keep the brain cells healthy. Reflexology stimulates the points on the foot corresponding to the brain and opens blocked energy passages and improves blood circulation, all of which contribute to brain activity. And of course, regular sessions will assuage unnecessary worry and panic over memory loss.

GOOD STEPS: FOR IMPROVING MEMORY

Each session should last 15 to 20 minutes and be done once a day.

1. Relax both feet with relaxation techniques, and end by a thumb press on the solar plexus point in both feet. Relax each foot separately.

2. Thumb walk up the five zones of one foot and work the points suggested below.

3. Thumb walk up the five zones of the other foot and work the points suggested below.

4. Integrate relaxation techniques throughout the session as needed to help your partner relax when you encounter tender spots.

REFLEX AREA	TECHNIQUE	RATIONALE
BRAIN	Finger roll	• Stimulate neural integration • Stimulate area of brain responsible for memory
PITUITARY AND PINEAL	Hook & back-up	• Stimulate endocrine functions
LUNGS AND CHEST	Thumb walk across	• Relax muscles • Regulate heart function
LUNGS AND CHEST	Lung press	• Deepen breathing
THYROID AND PARATHYROIDS	Thumb walk across	• Regulate metabolism and calcium use
SPINE	Spinal twist	• Stretch spine
SPINE	Thumb walk up, down, and across	• Stimulate neural activity
SPINE	Rotate onto thumb	• Loosen and improve circulation to spine
ADRENALS	Rotate onto thumb	• Balance energy levels • Mineral balance (some feel memory is affected by mineral imbalance)

- Do relaxation techniques and thumb press on the solar plexus point in both feet, and end with breeze strokes.

Suggested Visualization:

Let your partner imagine a beautiful cut crystal globe filled with all her best memories. Encourage your partner to get closer and closer to the globe until she can see all the beautiful objects, scents, and sounds inside. Have your partner reach into the globe through a special door and pick up each object inside and experience it. Then let her envision her head surrounded in a beautiful, soft purple light that is opening and clearing silvery memory passages in the brain.

Reflexology can give a new lease on life to the older generation. Not only will it provide improved health and well-being, but it can give them a role to play in their families and communities. They can become healers and counselors to younger people—as well as to their peers—who can benefit from the wisdom and experience they have to share.

CHAPTER TEN

THE ACTIVE LIFE: REFLEXOLOGY AND ATHLETICS

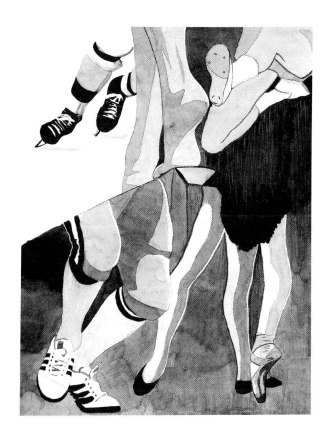

The word in sports is balance. For the professional marathoner as well as the weekend jogger, the key to peak athletic performance is keeping in balance. When athletes talk about being always on the fine edge, they mean the need to walk a fine line between extremes, for the athlete knows better than anyone how important it is for the body to be in peak condition, and that means cooperation among the various parts and systems of the body.

Consider muscles alone. Actually, muscles never are alone; they are distributed in groups throughout the body. Each set of muscles is balanced by another set. When one contracts, the other relaxes. In fact the electrochemical activity in any one muscle is a process of on and off, positive and negative, tension and release. Serious athletes work consistently on all muscle groups so that no one set dominates. For top performance, muscle groups must be uniformly developed and must function in harmony with one another.

Or consider the rhythms of exercise and practice. You can't exert yourself to the limit day after day. Professional athletes alternate periods of hard days with easy ones. After pushing the body hard in exercise and workouts, time out is needed to rest and let the tissue recover, because training is stressful. Each workout adds additional stress to the body so that it slowly builds up its endurance. No athlete thinks that the body can go the limit constantly. After a day of tough practice, the wise athlete schedules an "active rest day," one in which he or she will exercise but at a gentler and easier pace.

Competition involves balance, pitting your own talents and strengths against an opponent in the give-and-take of play, holding your own, meeting resistance, maintaining the balance until you find the advantage and overpower the other to score. And balance is important in team sports too. If you've ever been a member of a softball team or had a tennis partner, you know that throughout the game there are ever-shifting patterns of balance between fellow players. The common term for it is cooperation, but when you analyze the dynamics, it's a question of balance.

Balance in sports is physical, mental, emotional, and interpersonal. The physical body needs a balance of energies; emotions need to be kept in control so they work for you instead of against you; a cool head is required to keep advantages and disadvantages in perspective.

TRAINING

By making reflexology part of your regular training, you will be playing from the vantage point of strength and balance. One of my associates who is a marathon runner has a reflexology practice made up almost entirely of athletes. He finds that his clients play better, their times improve, their concentration is sharper, they suffer fewer injuries, and when they are injured they recover in much shorter time so they can return to their game. He recommends making reflexology a partner with other toning and stretching therapies and activities, such as massage and swimming, for general conditioning as well as recovery from sore and injured muscles.

Should you have a reflexology session immediately before competition? It depends. Serious and professional athletes shouldn't be too loose and relaxed before a game. Staying psyched up requires a certain amount of tension and flow of adrenaline. Sports counselors would suggest that for competitive athletes reflexology should be given about two days before, not on the day of the big event. Runners in the New York City Marathon who receive reflexology prefer it one to two days before the race. For amateur and weekend sports enthusiasts, however, who compete for fun rather than for living, that competitive tension isn't quite so important. For them, a little reflexology earlier in the day could be just the thing to help them unwind from their normal living activities and get ready for their event. However you incorporate it, reflexology should make you feel less tired and heavy after a game or race.

One of my clients is a competitive tennis player who often represents her country club in statewide tournaments. When she turned forty, she began suffering from tennis elbow, a painful condition that plagues many players, and had to receive cortisone shots. Needless to say, she also suffered anxiety in thinking that this meant she was over the hill and unable to play competitively again. She came to me for reflexology, and a couple of sessions eliminated most of the severe pain. Eventually she began competing again, always sure to schedule a session with me preceding an important match. In addition to working the neck, shoulder, spine, and arm areas on the foot, I paid special attention to working the adrenals, hoping they could be stimulated into producing their own cortisone. In time, she was able to dispense with her cortisone shots altogether.

Remember: before each routine in this chapter, set up the environment as described in Chapter Three. Prepare the materials needed such as lotion, towel, and cornstarch. Create the appropriate mood with lighting and music. Review the person's health history. Check the feet for cuts, bruises, sores, corns, or calluses. If necessary, clean the feet with a warm washcloth or handiwipe. Clear and center yourself.

GOOD STEPS: FOR REFLEXOLOGY BEFORE A GAME OR WORKOUT

Each session should last 20 minutes and be scheduled 2 to 3 hours before playing. For general conditioning, schedule 2 or 3 sessions per week.

1.   Relax both feet with relaxation techniques, and end by a thumb press on the solar plexus point in both feet. Relax each foot separately.

2.   Thumb walk up the five zones of one foot and work the points suggested below.

3.   Thumb walk up the five zones of the other foot and work the points suggested below.

4.   Integrate relaxation techniques throughout the session as needed to help your partner relax when you encounter tender spots.

REFLEX AREA	TECHNIQUE	RATIONALE
LUNGS/HEART/CHEST	Thumb walk	• Deepen breathing • Send oxygen to cells • Improve circulation
DIAPHRAGM	Thumb walk and rotate onto thumb	• Increase circulation and respiration
LUNGS AND CHEST	Lung press	• Relax chest • Regulate breathing

THYROID AND PARATHYROID	Thumb walk across	• Help balance metabolic rate • Help balance calcium and phosphate levels
BRAIN	Roll and rock	• Improve clarity of thought • Improve reception of sensory input
LIVER	Thumb walk diagonally across	• Blood production functions • Assist elimination of toxins • Balance blood pressure
KIDNEYS	Thumb walk and rotate onto thumb	• Help release of fluids • Help elimination of toxins • Balance blood pressure
ADRENALS	Thumb walk and rotate onto thumb	• Produce epinephrine for more energy
SPINE	Thumb walk up, down, and across	• Improve flexibility • Improve neural control over muscular activity
	Rotate onto thumb and spinal twist	• Clear nerve impulses
HIP/KNEE/LEG TRIANGLE	Finger walk	• Loosen and relax muscles
ENTIRE FOOT	Foot rocking	• Relax foot and leg

•   Do relaxation techniques and thumb press on the solar plexus point in both feet, and end with breeze strokes.

Suggested Visualization:

Let your partner imagine being on the court or in the gym, relaxed, alert, poised, energetic. Then have him see and feel himself playing a great, enjoyable game or experiencing a great, energizing workout.

Reflexology is also great after a workout or a heavy day of exercise and training when you feel stressed-out mentally and physically. Reflexology brings you back into balance. Of course, you may have to adjust the treatment depending on the sensitivity of your feet. Some athletes say that their feet kill them after a workout or a game. In this case, work the soreness out first with the easy relaxation exercises that should begin each reflexology session. Later you can work more deeply. Even though reflexology is not massage therapy, many athletes and sports people think of it as massage and look forward to it after a game or workout.

GOOD STEPS: FOR REFLEXOLOGY AFTER A GAME OR WORKOUT

Each session should last 20 minutes and follow your regular postgame shower.

1.   Relax both feet with relaxation techniques, and end by a thumb press on the solar plexus point in both feet. Relax each foot separately.

2.   Thumb walk up the five zones of one foot and work the points suggested below.

3.   Thumb walk up the five zones of the other foot and work the points suggested below.

4.   Integrate relaxation techniques throughout the session as needed to help your partner relax when you encounter tender spots.

REFLEX AREA	TECHNIQUE	RATIONALE
LUNG AND CHEST REGION (EMPHASIS ON SHOULDERS)	Thumb walk back and forth across	• Relax the upper torso • Deepen breathing
LUNGS AND CHEST	Lung press	• Relax chest region • Regulate breathing
DIAPHRAGM	Thumb walk and rotate onto thumb	• Relax muscle
ADRENALS	Thumb walk and rotate onto thumb	• Increased energy • Mineral balance
PANCREAS	Thumb walk across	• Balance blood sugar levels
SPINE	Thumb walk up, down, and across	• Release strain on back muscles
HIP/KNEE/LEG TRIANGLE	Finger walk	• Relax and bring circulation to these areas
SCIATIC NERVE ON INSIDE OF LEG, ACROSS THE BOTTOM OF THE HEEL, ON THE OUTSIDE OF THE FOOT BEHIND THE ANKLE	Thumb walk down, finger walk up	• Stimulate the energy flow and prevent blockage

•   Do relaxation techniques and thumb press on the solar plexus point in both feet, and end with breeze strokes.

Suggested Visualization:

Let your partner imagine she is lying on a bed of soft, aromatic pine needles in a pine forest.

MUSCLES

In addition to supplying muscle cells with nutrients and oxygen, the blood stream removes the toxins and waste products generated by increased muscle activity. During exercise, the bloodstream delivers only a minimal amount of nutrition to the muscles. If a muscle uses all its available energy, or if an inadequate amount of oxygen is available for complete energy use, waste products build up inside the muscle. Eventually these waste products will impede the muscle's ability to contract. This is why serious athletes will not work out strenuously two days in a row but alternate heavy workout days with easier ones. Enhanced circulation facilitates the removal of waste products from the body and prevents many of the aches, pains, spasms, and cramps that typically follow extended exercise periods.

GOOD STEPS: FOR TONING MUSCLES

Each session should last 30 minutes and be performed 2 to 3 times per week.

1.   Relax both feet with relaxation techniques, and end by a thumb press on the solar plexus point in both feet. Relax each foot separately.

2.   Thumb walk up the five zones of one foot and work the points suggested below.

3.   Thumb walk up the five zones of the other foot and work the points suggested below.

4.   Integrate relaxation techniques throughout the session as needed to help your partner relax when you encounter tender spots.

Give a complete session with extra relaxation techniques to serve as an overall toner. Thumb press on the solar plexus point in both feet, and end with breeze strokes. A reflexology session is a perfect companion for any physical workout.

Suggested Visualization:

Let your partner see each muscle group in the body as supple, long, and strong. Encourage him to see his body in its ideal state, and to feel how it moves during sports, or while dancing with a favorite partner. If you like, listen to your partner's favorite workout music during the session.

Muscle injuries may involve overstretching or tearing of muscle fibers. Tears create scar tissue, which is more fibrous and tighter than uninjured tissue. Blood does not flow well through scar tissue. Reflexology can assist the delivery of blood to those areas of the body that need it most. A sufficient supply of blood is necessary for oxygen to reach each cell. Muscles will work at their peak efficiency only if the cell environment is properly supplied with oxygen, nutrients, and other vital minerals, enzymes, and hormones. Without the free flow of blood throughout the body, muscles cannot contract and relax as smoothly or as strongly as they are required to do during vigorous exercise.

GOOD STEPS: FOR MUSCLE INJURIES

Each session should last 15 to 20 minutes and be done 2 or 3 times per week.

1. Relax both feet with relaxation techniques, and end by a thumb press on the solar plexus point in both feet. Relax each foot separately.

2. Thumb walk up the five zones of one foot and work the points suggested below.

3. Thumb walk up the five zones of the other foot and work the points suggested below.

4. Integrate relaxation techiques throughout the session as needed to help your partner relax when you encounter tender spots.

REFLEX AREA	TECHNIQUE	RATIONALE
AREA RELATED TO INJURED MUSCLES	Thumb or finger walk	• Relax specific musculature
LUNGS AND CHEST	Thumb or finger walk vertically up zones and across	• Improve circulation to heal affected area • Open breathing • Help relax
ADRENALS	Rotate onto thumb	• Stimulate anti-inflammatory hormones • Improve muscle tone
SPINE	Thumb walk up, down, and across	• Relax all back muscles
LYMPHATIC NECK/CHEST/GROIN	Finger walk	• Carry away waste from inflammatory process
REFERRAL AREA FOR THE INJURED MUSCLES	Work (if appropriate)	• Help balance energy and improve circulation throughout same zone

• Do relaxation techniques and thumb press on the solar plexus point in both feet, and end with breeze strokes.

Suggested Visualization:

Ask your partner to see the injured muscle as a ripped or knotted piece of pink silk. Have her gently knit together the fibers of the fabric, or gently unravel the knot until the fabric is a single loose, strong, and supple swatch once again.

INJURIES

It's been said that the single greatest factor in athletic improvement is to remain free of injuries. You know how being injured can set you back. Not only can you not play, you lose training time, you can't exercise, and when you do return, you can't just pick up where you left off. Often the injury will result in residual soreness or a weakened condition that could affect your game adversely for the rest of your life. All serious athletes have some type of residual soreness and most learn how to live with it, but reflexology can eliminate much of it altogether.

There is no hard proof as to why athletes who receive reflexology have fewer injuries, but it seems to make sense that if the body is balanced and functioning well and your concentration is more finely tuned, you should be able to prevent the more common types of injuries that result from poor judgment or playing when you're not physically up to it. We know people tend to sleep better, feel more rested, and consequently have more energy for whatever they plan to do when they receive reflexology on a regular basis. There is also strong evidence that people who do things to take care of themselves, such as reflexology, meditation, or some form of exercise, have a more concerned attitude toward their bodies, monitor themselves more closely, watch their movements, and refrain from pushing themselves too hard, and consequently prevent injuries.

GOOD STEPS: FOR MENDING BROKEN BONES

Each session should last 10 minutes and be done once a day. Be careful not to manipulate the area that is broken.

1. Relax both feet with relaxation techniques, and end by a thumb press on the solar plexus point in both feet. Relax each foot separately.

2. Thumb walk up the five zones of one foot and work the points suggested below.

3. Thumb walk up the five zones of the other foot and work the points suggested below.

4.   Integrate relaxation techniques throughout the session as needed to help your partner relax when you encounter tender spots.

REFLEX AREA	TECHNIQUE	RATIONALE
AREA RELATIVE TO THE BROKEN BONE	Thumb or finger walk	• Facilitate proper healing of the specific bone
HEART/CHEST/ LUNG AREA	Thumb or finger walk	• Improve circulation to injured area
LUNGS AND CHEST	Lung press	• Relax and regulate breathing
THYROID AND PARATHYROIDS	Thumb walk	• Regulate calcium levels
ADRENALS	Rotate onto thumb	• Help reduce inflammation and facilitate healing • Produce hormones involved with mineral balance
REFERRAL AREA FOR THE INJURY	Thumb or finger walk	• Working the body part that corresponds to the injury and is in the same zone will help facilitate healing

•   Do relaxation techniques and thumb press on the solar plexus point in both feet, and end with breeze strokes.

Suggested Visualization:

Let your partner imagine that a strong, thick golden rope is running through the broken bone, coaxing the broken pieces to heal together again. Let your partner actually see the pieces of bone mending together in whatever images are most powerful for him.

REFLEXOLOGY AND SLEEP

Everyone needs time out for relaxation, but this is especially true of an athlete, whose performance depends on coordination of mind and body. Being physically and mentally alert and fit is of utmost importance in winning the game. Often athletes, even amateurs, will not sleep well the night before an important game. Fortunately, studies have shown that missing your usual forty winks the night before is not as detrimental as you might suppose. What's more important is that you rest. Sleep and rest are not synonymous. We all know that it's possible to sleep all night yet wake up in the morning feeling worn out because we didn't sleep soundly or restfully. If you can't sleep because of a competition on the next day, you can still perform well if you manage to rest during the night, in spite of being sleepless. Athletes who receive reflexology report that they sleep more soundly, and that they rest well in a relaxed state, even on the occasional nights when they can't get to sleep.

KEEPING YOUR MIND'S EYE ON THE BALL

"Keep your eye on the ball" is advice that has leaped from the sports arena into every walk of life. It means: stay focused, concentrate, keep your mind on what you're doing. Reflexology has helped people keep their eyes "on the ball" at work and play so that they perform more efficiently. Not only is their attention more finely tuned, but their *intention* is stronger also. When they set goals, they meet them. They know what they want to achieve and they do it. For example, an athlete who wants to work on weight loss or a backhand swing or train for a specific race can keep her attention and willpower focused on those goals.

One of the latest techniques in sports training is to keep your eye on the ball even before the game, even when you're not practicing. This form of visualization is used by more and more sports psychologists and coaches around the country to improve their players' performances in every field. Football players mentally rehearse every possible play, runners race the entire course step by step in their minds, racketball players spar with their opponents in their heads before they get out on the courts. It's been demonstrated in numerous studies that you can actually improve your game and performances by creatively visualizing them beforehand.

GOOD STEPS: FOR PREGAME VISUALIZATIONS

You can incorporate visualization into a reflexology session by seeing yourself in competition going through the physical and emotional movements of the game. Or spend the reflexology session with an open mind, thinking of nothing in particular and then use the time immediately afterward for serious visualization. The residual effects of reflexology will allow you to make better use of the visualization training whenever you engage in it, immediately afterward or later on.

In addition to the personal health benefits of reflexology, remember that reflexology operates on an interpersonal and social level as well. Just as it enhances relationships between couples, parents and children, friends and colleagues, it can be used by team members to get to know each other and show concern for each other's physical condition and performance level in a warm, relaxed way. It can nurture friendships on a soccer team or allow you to get to know your regular racketball partner in a way that can't be achieved just by the usual camaraderie on the playing field or in the locker room.

Increasing numbers of athletes are discovering that the "competitive edge" has a cooperative effect, using the best talents and strengths of the team members and the best training techniques; whether they come from sports medicine, nutritional programs, body work, or the many psychological and spiritual methodologies available today. Reflexology should be one of the many paths which teach the athlete that excellence and the ultimate self-challenge do not always mean going it alone.

The body is like a pond and it should never become stagnant. This goes for everyone, athletes and nonathletes alike. We each have a certain level of activity in our lives to which our bodies grow accustomed. When that activity is curtailed for any reason, such as illness or a busy work schedule that doesn't allow time for exercise, the body becomes a stagnant pond. It needs stirring up. Juices need to flow and circulate. The body depends on the flow of oxygen, minerals, and other nutrients for normal daily living and especially for vigorous athletic activity. Reflexology is an easy and enjoyable way to keep those juices flowing, to maintain the proper balances within the body, and to provide the energy you need for peak performances.

CHAPTER ELEVEN

GETTING UNHOOKED: OVERCOMING ADDICTIONS WITH REFLEXOLOGY

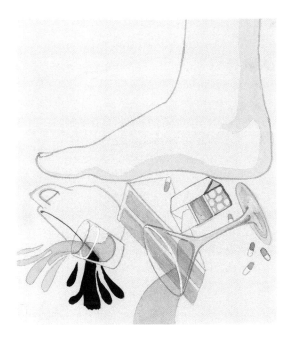

A fundamental fact about modern life is that stress and frustration are causing many Americans to become addicted to drugs and alcohol. But addictive behavior isn't just limited to "drunks and druggies" as many people believe. Tobacco, food, coffee, even work and shopping lend themselves to abuse. The lighthearted jokes about the incurable "chocoholic" who can sniff out a Hershey bar across town cover up a serious tendency to get hooked. Whether it's too many cups of coffee, too many cigarettes, daily shopping binges just to make ourselves feel good, or the extra hours of overtime we convince ourselves we have to put in at the office or workplace, as a nation we display rather serious addictive behaviors.

BREAKING THE HABIT

Breaking the habit is like breaking a lock: It requires the right combination. In this case, it can depend on the length of the addiction, the specific plan or therapy for kicking the habit, support from family and friends, the refusal to tolerate accomplices who encourage the habit, and commitment. Without a strong determination to get well, addictions persist. In fact, one's intention to get over an addiction is probably the single most important factor in beginning a program to replace the addictive patterns in your life with healthy, nonaddictive patterns of living. All of these are the traditional keys for getting unhooked. But today there is another therapy being used in drug and alcohol rehabilitation programs—reflexology.

Reflexology can take the place of addictive behavior because it is an alternate activity with some of the same characteristics as addiction but without the negative impact. Reflexology junkies? Sort of.

Addictive behavior is engaged in both as a form of reward and as an escape. Reflexology is also both reward and escape but without the calories, the hangover, the crash, or the jitters. It is a safe form of rewarding yourself, pampering yourself when you feel down, giving yourself a healthful and wonderful high. It is also an escape in the best sense of that word. Let's face it, there's a lot in modern life that we should escape from now and then— traffic jams, sirens, crowds, deadlines, overwork, even the incessant chatter going on inside our heads! Slipping into a relaxed state through reflexology is all you need to drop out for an hour or so, to clear your mind and steady your nerves so you can deal more effectively with the problems and aggravations you have to face. The meditative quality of reflexology is good for the soul, and as Alcoholics Anonymous supporters remind us, addictions are as much a spiritual as a physical affliction.

One way to look at it is that people begin to love themselves in a wholesome way. And this is crucial for breaking addictions. There are many theories about how and why people become addicted, but a common explanation is that addictions are basically self-destructive behavior, arising from self-hatred. Certainly, a full-blown addiction displays plenty of self-hatred and self-destruction, even hatred and destruction aimed outward toward others. When people admit to themselves that they can't make it without resorting to drink or drugs, they simply reinforce the image they have of themselves as weak, unlovable, and self-destructive individuals. Feelings of weakness, shame, and guilt begin to escalate. A vicious cycle develops that frequently results in abusive behavior to others who get pulled into it.

ALCOHOL AND DRUG ABUSE

In New Jersey a graduate of my professional training course has been working in an alcohol and drug rehabilitation center. He uses reflexology on many of the clients in the program and has discovered that regular sessions eliminate much of the edginess and anxiety caused by substance deprivation. Clients improve much more rapidly and often without the harmful effects of the additional stress that giving up one's crutch can cause.

Remember: before each routine in this chapter, set up the environment as described in Chapter Three. Prepare the materials needed such as lotion, towel, and cornstarch. Create the appropriate mood with lighting and music. Review the person's health history. Check the feet for cuts, bruises, sores, corns, or calluses. If necessary, clean the feet with a warm washcloth or handiwipe. Clear and center yourself.

GOOD STEPS: FOR ALCOHOL AND DRUG ABUSE

Each session should last 15 to 20 minutes and be done whenever you feel a craving, or at least twice a week.

1.   Relax both feet with relaxation techniques, and end by a thumb press on the solar plexus point in both feet. Relax each foot separately.

2.   Thumb walk up the five zones of one foot and work the points suggested below.

3.   Thumb walk up the five zones of the other foot and work the points suggested below.

4.   Integrate relaxation techniques throughout the session as needed to help your partner relax when you encounter tender spots.

REFLEX AREA	TECHNIQUE	RATIONALE
CHEST/LUNG/ BRONCHIALS/ DIAPHRAGM	Thumb walk	• Help relax and free breathing
THYROID	Thumb walk	• Balance metabolism
PITUITARY AND PINEAL	Hook & back-up	• Stimulate all glands • Produce melatonin for mood elevation
HYPOTHALAMUS	Hook & back-up	• Balance emotional stress
BRAIN	Finger roll	• Help the brain function without the need for alcohol or drugs
PANCREAS	Thumb walk	• Regulate blood sugar
LIVER	Thumb walk diagonally (crosshatching)	• Purify the bloodstream and filter wastes
INTESTINES	Thumb walk diagonally across	• Activate elimination of toxins • Absorption of nutrients
BLADDER AND KIDNEYS	Thumb walk and rotate onto thumb	• Eliminate wastes and toxins • Ease fluid retention
ADRENALS	Thumb walk	• Improve energy • Balance moods

- Do relaxation techniques and thumb press on the solar plexus point in both feet, and end with breeze strokes.

Suggested Visualization:

Let your partner imagine he is a king (or favorite role model) sitting on a beautiful purple throne, feeling his full power and compassion. Next, have your partner see all his subjects and loved ones surrounding him and gazing at him with support. Then, have him imagine himself ruling the kingdom of his own life wisely and well.

Or, let your partner imagine she is standing on a mountaintop and watching the most beautiful pink sunrise she has ever seen.

QUITTING SMOKING ONCE AND FOR ALL

If you've ever quit or known anyone who has tried to quit smoking, you know about the periods of intolerable craving for a cigarette. Withdrawal from nicotine can cause people to climb the walls. It's suddenly clear to them just how important a cigarette is in their lives and just how dependent upon cigarettes they are. Reflexology won't prevent all the tingles in the mouth that demand a cigarette, but it can temper the side effects of nervousness, anxiety, and irritability that accompany withdrawal pains.

A client of mine who was a heavy smoker told me after each session that reflexology made him appreciate his body more and that he felt so good afterward that it seemed wrong to pollute it with another cigarette.

GOOD STEPS: FOR QUITTING SMOKING

Each session should last 15 to 20 minutes and be done twice a week or whenever you feel the urge to smoke.

1. Relax both feet with relaxation techniques, and end by a thumb press on the solar plexus point in both feet. Relax each foot separately.

2. Thumb walk up the five zones of one foot and work the points suggested below.

3. Thumb walk up the five zones of the other foot and work the points suggested below.

4. Integrate relaxation techniques throughout the session as needed to help your partner relax when you encounter tender spots.

REFLEX AREA	TECHNIQUE	RATIONALE
LUNGS AND CHEST	Thumb walk across	• Improve and normalize breathing for better delivery of oxygen to tissue
LUNGS AND CHEST	Lung press	• Relax chest muscles • Deepen breathing
DIAPHRAGM LINE	Thumb walk back and forth across	• Relax breathing muscles
DIAPHRAGM	Rotate onto thumb	• Clear tension in chest area
HEART AREA	Thumb walk	• Clear nicotine-constricted blood vessels
SHOULDER AREA ON FRONT AND BACK OF FOOT	Thumb walk	• Bring circulation to area • Relax shoulders and free up breathing
NECK	Hang on ridge	• Stimulate circulation to neck, throat, and thyroid
THYROID AND THROAT	Thumb walk	• Balance metabolism and relax throat
PITUITARY AND PINEAL HYPOTHALAMUS	Hook & back-up	• Boost energy levels • Balance hormonal function • Elevate mood
SPINE (ESPECIALLY THORACIC)	Thumb walk up, down, and across	• Stimulate spinal nerves to chest
UPPER BACK AREAS ON FRONT OF FOOT	Thumb walk	• Open up lungs
LIVER	Thumb walk diagonally across	• Detoxify blood

| KIDNEY | Thumb walk | • Facilitate elimination of waste through urine (people experience increased urination when nicotine is taken away) |
| ADRENALS | Thumb walk and rotate onto thumb | • Energy balance
• Mineral balance |

• Do relaxation techniques and thumb press on the solar plexus point in both feet, and end with breeze strokes.

Suggested Visualization:

Have your partner visualize his breath as golden light. Each time he inhales, he also inhales the power and will to stop smoking. Each time he exhales, he exhales a little bit of the need to smoke.

LOSING WEIGHT

Clients who use reflexology along with a diet to lose weight say they feel so good after a session that they want to watch what they eat the rest of the day and not lose the feeling by bolting down another soda or Twinkie. It's this kind of appreciation for one's body that reflexology brings so easily and naturally. And it feels wonderful. You get the experience yourself without the abused substance. You can learn how to feel great without martinis, marijuana, or M&Ms.

The vicious cycle of feeling bad about yourself and then using a harmful substance as a reward to feel better seems especially true for those trying to lose weight. They begin with a poor self-image of being fat. Finally they realize that something's got to be done about it, so they either try to stay away from fattening foods or they plunge into a "surefire" diet guaranteed to take off "ugly inches." But each time they fail to stick to it, they feel all the more miserable. Each failure reinforces their negative self-image. Eventually they end up either hating themselves outright or holding themselves in very low esteem. Then to make themselves feel better they resort to the only remedy they know: food.

The real remedy, of course, is love. They need to learn how to love themselves in a healthy and constructive manner. They need to feel good about themselves so they know they are worthy of their own love. Reflexology is precisely that. It is a good reward system that makes you feel great without any negative side effects. So learn to pick up your foot, rather than a fork!

A client of mine referred to herself as a "diet junkie" since she claimed to have tried all the diets and consulted all the diet doctors, to no avail. Finally a complete physical examination revealed a glandular imbalance which affected her weight and her emotions. She was on a regular roller-coaster ride of overeating, gaining weight, feeling bad about herself, and assuaging her depression by more eating. Reflexology, however, made her feel good physically, and the two or three sessions each week gave her the nurturing through touch that she had been seeking through food. Because she began to feel better all over, she decided to watch her diet more carefully and even started exercising. While she will never be as pencil-thin as a fashion model, she has slimmed down considerably. What's even better, though, is that she now leads a much more balanced life and is generally experiencing a state of good health that she never realized was possible for her.

GOOD STEPS: FOR LOSING WEIGHT

Each session should last about 15 minutes and be done every day whenever you feel a craving for food other than at approved times for meals.

1.   Relax both feet with relaxation techniques, and end by a thumb press on the solar plexus point in both feet. Relax each foot separately.

2.   Thumb walk up the five zones of one foot and work the points suggested below.

3.   Thumb walk up the five zones of the other foot and work the points suggested below.

4.   Integrate relaxation techniques throughout the session as needed to help your partner relax when you encounter tender spots.

REFLEX AREA	TECHNIQUE	RATIONALE
STOMACH	Thumb walk across	• Stimulate production and release of digestive juices • Smooth muscle activity
PANCREAS	Thumb walk across	• Regulate blood sugar level • Stimulate production and release of digestive juices
LIVER	Thumb walk	• Produce bile • Store and release glycogen
GALLBLADDER	Rotate onto thumb and pivot	• Release bile that breaks down fat and assist in elimination of waste
INTESTINES	Thumb walk diagonally	• Absorption of nutrients • Elimination of wastes
KIDNEYS AND BLADDER	Thumb walk and rotate onto thumb	• Fluid elimination • Kidneys secrete hormones involved with protein and carbohydrate metabolism • Mineral balance
ADRENALS	Rotate onto thumb and thumb walk	• Improve energy
THYROID	Thumb walk across	• Regulate metabolism
NECK/THYROID	Toe rotation	• Stimulate thyroid
PITUITARY	Hook & back-up	• Stimulate proper functioning of all glands
HYPOTHALAMUS	Hook & back-up	• Control appetite
NECK AND HEAD	Toe boogie	• Free blockage imbalance in thyroid

•   Do relaxation techniques and thumb press on the solar plexus point in both feet, and end with breeze strokes.

Suggested Visualization:

First, let your partner see herself at perfect weight. Have her develop the image in as much detail as possible. Then, encourage your partner to see every inhalation as loving pink light, and to breathe out a little of the need to overeat each time she exhales.

BUDDY UP!

When reflexology is given by a friend or family member, it becomes a sociable way of being loved and pampered by someone who is important to you, someone whose love and attention can help support your commitment to a diet or a no-drinking plan. To break the destructive cycle of hate and self-pity we need to create a constructive cycle of love and support. So often teenagers will smoke, drink, or use drugs precisely because they feel no one understands or loves them. Peer pressure (from equally miserable adolescents) rounds out the vicious circle. Everywhere a teenager looks there is opportunity and encouragement to engage in pseudo-loving behavior—a cigarette, a beer, a joint of marijuana, another candy bar. Reflexology can break the cycle by creating relationships among close friends in which love, appreciation, and esteem are expressed in a healthful, nonverbal way when you find it difficult to express yourself in words.

GOOD STEPS: FOR STICKING TO YOUR PLAN OF REFORM

Find someone to give you reflexology whom you can trust and who has a sincere interest in your reform program. If your buddy doesn't know reflexology, teach him yourself and let him read this book. Then on a calendar, schedule reflexology sessions at a time when they will be convenient for both of you. This may seem overly simple, but it's little commitments like this that will keep you faithful.

THREE WAYS TO USE REFLEXOLOGY TO OVERCOME ADDICTIVE BEHAVIOR

First, use it as a diversion if at all possible. Instead of mixing a scotch and water at the end of a busy day, do reflexology when you get home. If it would not be too disruptive at the office, slip off your shoe and work your foot for a few minutes while you sit at your desk instead of going for another cup of coffee or a cigarette. On a Saturday afternoon when you have nothing to do but go shopping for all those things you know you don't really need, schedule a mutual reflexology get-together with a friend. It's a better bargain than you'll find in the mall! However you are able to manage it, try to grab your foot and work even just a few areas. Simple reflexology techniques can calm a craving.

Second, plan one, two, or three sessions into every week. Don't just make a halfhearted intention to do this. Write it on your calendar. Make an "appointment" with your spouse, a friend, or a neighbor who can do it for you. Stick to this routine. One of my clients always gets off the table at the end of every session and says, "Ah, that fix will hold me for three days!" Of course, there's no formula for how much reflexology will provide the right fix for any individual or for how many days it will hold. But my client is right in that when you begin to look forward to reflexology every week or more often, it becomes a kind of fix in your cycle of work and play. You anticipate it and know that you'll feel good. You gain confidence in waiting for it. And you actually start to feel better in general just thinking about it.

Third, there is a cumulative effect to regular reflexology sessions. Again, there is no timetable or system of measurement to say how it will work for you, but you will experience your own ongoing high that will build up as reflexology begins to work on the various levels of your life. Physically you will feel much better. Mentally you'll be more alert and creative. Emotionally you'll be on a more even keel. In general, you'll find yourself handling life better and more successfully, including your plan for kicking your habit, which, as the experts tell us, may take time. Overcoming addictions is an ongoing commitment.

WHY DOES REFLEXOLOGY HELP?

How reflexology manages to do all this is still something of a mystery. Studies, however, have shown that alcoholics, for example, do not produce enough endorphins, the hormones that block pain and are associated with feeling good and energetic. Reflexology assists the body in producing endorphins. People who pump drugs into their bodies suffer from all types of chemical and glandular imbalances. As they slowly withdraw, their bodies experience even more upsetting imbalances. Reflexology helps the various systems of the body to come back into balance.

The metabolisms of people who are overweight run amuck both from having to manage the excess weight and from what might be a diet of junk food. Reflexology helps the metabolism function properly. Furthermore, many people suffer serious physical damage resulting from their addictions. Liver damage among alcoholics is a case in point. Reflexology can assist the body in repairing itself. Last of all, men and women who pollute their bodies with caffeine, nicotine, junk food, alcohol, and other drugs have considerable amounts of toxic substances in their bloodstreams. Reflexology can assist rehabilitation programs by helping to eliminate impurities.

The most important element in kicking any habit is willpower, the intention and commitment to make it work. You can improve your life and health if you really want to, but it takes more than just a few casual resolutions. We all know people who are going to start dieting tomorrow or give up cigarettes after exams or cut down on drinking as soon as the holidays are over. Tomorrow never comes and holidays (fortunately and unfortunately!) are always coming. And so these people never quit. Successfully breaking the habit means making up your mind to do so and then making up a plan that will help you do it. It also means not becoming discouraged if you fail now and then. Someone once said that there is no failure in falling down; the real failure is to fall down and not get back up. Reflexology can literally help us get back up on our feet by making us more aware of ourselves and stronger in our commitments. It works fast. One session can prove to you that you really can change. You can feel good without abusing food, drink, or drugs.

While it is not a panacea, reflexology can be the vehicle for pulling together all the various components of rehabilitation. It is a reward system, a detoxifier, a time to be supported in your decision by someone who loves you, a diversion, and a way to focus your energy on the things that are really important in your life. And most of all, it is a way of showing yourself that you really do love being just who you are.

CHAPTER TWELVE

THE FINAL STEPS: REFLEXOLOGY AND TERMINAL ILLNESS

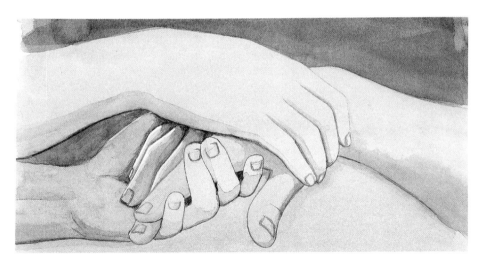

We live in an age of slow death. People's dying lingers. The end is repeatedly postponed. This is partially due to our diagnosing terminal illness earlier and our ability to prolong life with drugs and life-supportive technology. But we also live in an age plagued by terminal illness, the various cancers and AIDS-related diseases being the most devastating.

Reflexology can be an important therapy to make the final days, weeks, or months as comfortable as possible. My coauthor used reflexology on a friend who was dying of an AIDS-related pneumonia in a New York hospital. The dying man, an Episcopal priest, was unable to speak or communicate naturally in the final two months of life due to an oxygen mask that tightly covered his nose and mouth. Visits by his family and friends were strained and lacked the lively dialogue that had characterized his relationships when he was well. Reflexology offered a way to communicate silently, express love and concern, and help the man relax. He often fell into a deep sleep shortly after the first relaxation techniques. Working the points for the chest area, especially with the lung press, often coincided with a steadier, more comfortable breathing. On waking he always said that, since he entered the hospital, his best and soundest sleep occurred when his feet were being worked.

Health care professionals who work with the dying and their families notice that there is a spontaneous tendency among even close friends and family members to stop touching the patient, sometimes as soon as he or she is diagnosed as having a terminal illness. It seems this has little to do with the fear of contagion, and more to do with a natural urge not to want to touch the dead—as if the diagnosis itself were the same as signing the death certificate. Reflexology provides a systematic way to touch the dying, which is therapeutic for them as well as for their friends and visitors. It gives a reason for visiting. It offers something positive to do. It takes the mind off the suffering and focuses it on relaxation and feeling better.

While laying on of hands is always beneficial for the terminally ill, at times it may not be possible to touch them directly where the pain is, either because it is internal or because the body cannot tolerate pressure there. The feet are seldom in too much pain to be worked; and because the entire body is represented on the foot, reflexology sessions can directly influence internal organs and painful areas of the body.

From the earlier chapters in the book, select the Good Steps appropriate to the person you are working on, considering the nature of the illness as well as the person's psychological frame of mind. Routines that are generally helpful in most instances are:

to boost the immune system . . . page 144
to overcome fatigue . . . page 135
to nurture your partner . . . page 161
for someone confined to bed . . . page 209
for edema . . . page 235
for ovarian/breast cysts or growths . . . page 177

CHAPTER THIRTEEN

USING REFLEXOLOGY TO STRENGTHEN THE BODY'S SYSTEMS

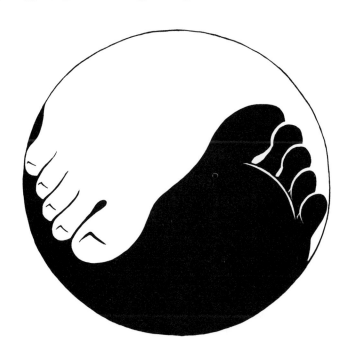

I have mentioned throughout this book that the body functions as a whole, and I have described the major organs and glands that make up the whole body. We are as healthy as the weakest of our glands and organs. As we bring new vitality and increased function to an organ or gland, the whole body feels stronger and healthier.

Many of the organs and glands unite to form a system in the body. This means they work interdependently to achieve their function. The names of these systems are as follows:

1.	Nervous system	6.	Respiratory system
2.	Muscular system	7.	Digestive system
3.	Skeletal system	8.	Urinary system
4.	Circulatory system	9.	Endocrine system
5.	Lymphatic system	10.	Reproductive system

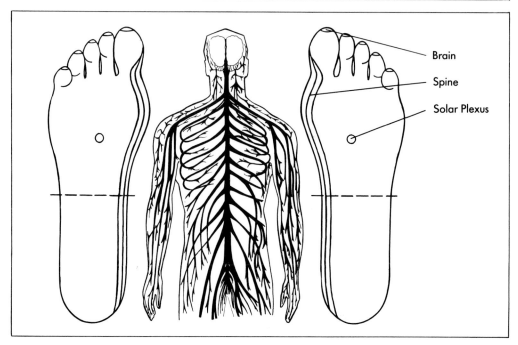

Brain

Spine

Solar Plexus

1. THE NERVOUS SYSTEM

The nervous system is comprised of the central nervous system, including the brain and spinal cord; the peripheral nervous system, including the autonomic nervous system; and the solar plexus. The function of the nervous system is to relay communication from the brain to all parts of the body and to bring communication from all parts of the body to the brain.

The solar plexus reflex helps to calm and relax the entire nervous system.

The brain reflex points on the foot are located in the big toe. The spinal cord has its reflexes along the spine area of the foot. The reflex area for the peripheral nervous system—the nerves that radiate out to all the organs and glands—is located along the spine reflex area but closer to the sole of the foot than the actual spine.

The brain is divided into several areas that have developed chronologically as mankind has evolved. The oldest part of the brain, the *brain stem,* controls all the vital life functions: respiration, blood pressure, pulse rate, and alertness. The brain stem's reflex point is at the base of the ball of the big toe. Right above this is the reflex point for the *cerebellum,* which regulates sleep, crude consciousness, breathing, and circulation, and coordinates movement and balance. Above this area in the big toe is the area of the pituitary, pineal gland, thalamus, and hypothalamus. Above this is the area for the *cerebral cortex (cerebrum),* which is the most recently evolved part of the brain and which comprises seventy percent of the brain. The cerebral cortex is divided into right and left hemispheres, which together control all our higher senses and functions—refined movement, consciousness, and communication skills. The left hemisphere, whose reflex points are on the left big toe, governs the right side of the body as well as speech, language, writing, logic, mathematical abilities, and analytic thinking. The right hemisphere, whose reflex points are on the right big toe, governs the left side of the body, as well as spatial relationships, pattern perception, artistic creativity, and intuitive and nonverbal understanding.

Thus to improve the functions associated with one of the brain hemispheres, we would work that big toe!

Remember: before each routine in this chapter, set up the environment as described in Chapter Three. Prepare the materials needed such as lotion, towel, and cornstarch. Create the appropriate mood with lighting and music.

Review the person's health history. Check the feet for cuts, bruises, sores, corns, or calluses. If necessary, clean the feet with a warm washcloth or handiwipe. Clear and center yourself.

GOOD STEPS: FOR THE NERVOUS SYSTEM

Each session should last 15 to 20 minutes and be done twice a week or whenever you feel the need.

1. Relax both feet with relaxation techniques, and end by a thumb press on the solar plexus point in both feet. Relax each foot separately.

2. Thumb walk up the five zones of one foot and work the points suggested below.

3. Thumb walk up the five zones of the other foot and work the points suggested below.

4. Integrate relaxation techniques throughout the session as needed to help your partner relax when you encounter tender spots.

REFLEX AREA	TECHNIQUE	RATIONALE
SPINE	Thumb walk and rotate	• Improve circulation and energy to central nervous system
SIDE OF SPINE (CLOSER TO SOLE)	Thumb walk and rotate	• Improve circulation and energy to peripheral nervous system
BRAIN	Finger roll	• Improve circulation and nerve conductivity
SOLAR PLEXUS	Thumb press	• Relax nervous system

• Do relaxation techniques and thumb press on the solar plexus point in both feet, and end with breeze strokes.

2. THE MUSCULAR SYSTEM

The muscular system includes all the muscles of the body. Muscles contract and relax to provide motion and maintain postural stability in the body. There are voluntary muscles, which we associate with conscious movement and involuntary muscles, which perform vital functions, such as the heart, diaphragm, and intestinal walls.

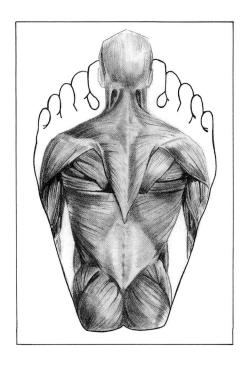

As we work the foot, we are contacting and strengthening every muscle in the body. Wherever you feel muscular tension, find the corresponding area on your foot and work that area until the tenderness begins to lessen. Find the area by using the grid map of the foot. For example, muscular tension just above the right shoulder blade would be at the top of the right foot below the toes at the same zone that the body feels the tension. Look for the tenderest area of the shoulder reflex to find the most effective reflex point.

SEE GOOD STEPS:

For Toning Muscles, page 248. For Muscle Injuries, page 249.

3. THE SKELETAL SYSTEM

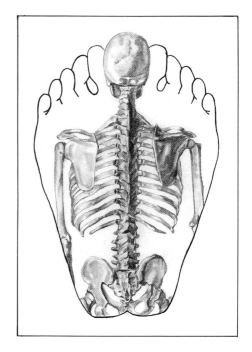

The skeletal system comprises all the bones in the body. Its function is to give structure and support, to protect internal organs and, along with the muscles, to allow movement of the body. It is also responsible for producing red blood cells for the circulatory system, and for storing minerals such as calcium, cobalt, and copper.

Please remember that we will also be affecting the muscles that connect to the bones we are working, so both the muscles and bones will be strengthened simultaneously.

SEE GOOD STEPS:

For Mending Broken Bones, page 251.

4. THE CIRCULATORY SYSTEM

The circulatory system contains the heart, blood vessels, and the blood. The arteries and capillaries carry fresh blood full of oxygen and nutrients to all the cells of the body. The veins carry blood full of carbon dioxide and waste products back to the heart and lungs for purification.

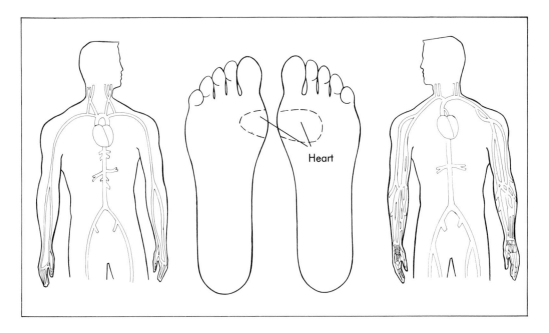

Heart

The circulatory system provides the cells with all they need for health and vitality. It carries oxygen, vitamins, minerals, hormones, and antibodies to where they are needed. If, because of stress, the cells are deprived of nutrition, oxygen, and the cleansing of waste products, then we have the first step toward disease.

To improve circulation, work the heart area, and then all areas of the foot to free the foot itself of obstructions to circulation and increase the circulation to all parts of the body.

SEE GOOD STEPS:

For High or Low Blood Pressure, page 149.
For Heart Problems, page 237.

5. THE LYMPHATIC SYSTEM

The lymphatic system is comprised of the lymph vessels and ducts, lymph nodes, lymph fluid, the spleen, tonsils, adenoids, thymus gland, and the appendix. Its function is to protect the body from infection and disease and to create immunity. The lymph vessels carry the interstitial fluids which bathe and detoxify all parts of the body back into the blood. The lymph nodes are found where the lymph vessels converge; they produce lymph cells and antibodies and filter out and destroy substances considered harmful to the body.

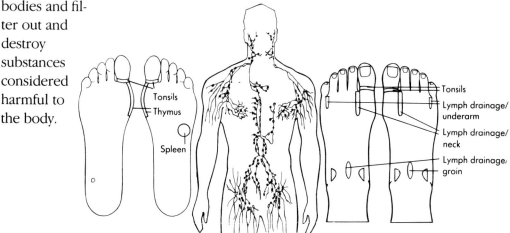

The tonsils are found at the back of the mouth and the adenoids are in the back of the nasal cavity. Both are specialized lymph nodes. The spleen is a mass of lymphoid tissue in which old and damaged cells and bacteria are filtered out. The spleen also stores iron from broken-down red blood cells, making this a good area to work in cases of anemia.

The thymus gland produces hormones which stimulate the production of lymphocytes and lymph tissue in children. Its role in adults is not yet fully understood, but it does play an important role in immune function with T lymphocytes, which secrete a substance that breaks down certain tumor and other foreign cells.

To strengthen the immune system and help the body to recover from colds and infections, we work the lymphatic reflexes on the foot and stimulate the spleen, tonsils, adenoids and thymus areas.

SEE GOOD STEPS:

For Boosting the Immune System, page 144.

6. THE RESPIRATORY SYSTEM

The respiratory system is made up of the nose, sinuses, and cilia, which filter the outside air; the larynx and vocal cords, which vibrate to produce sound; and the trachea, bronchial tubes, lungs, and diaphragm. The diaphragm is a muscle which is seventy-five percent responsible for the breathing process.

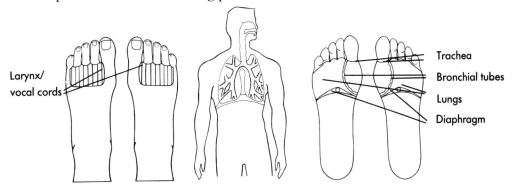

Larynx/vocal cords

Trachea
Bronchial tubes
Lungs
Diaphragm

The purpose of the respiratory system is to bring oxygen into the blood and to release carbon dioxide and unwanted gases back into the air. Every cell in the body is dependent on oxygen for its metabolism. Oxygen brought to the cell by the respiratory system and food brought to the cell by the digestive system combine to produce energy, or the fuel of life.

When breathing is shallow, the body tends to become toxic and acidic, and the muscles of the neck and shoulders tense. By opening the breathing, we open the emotions, and allow the whole body to feel oxygenated and vital.

Work all reflexes to the lungs on the ball of the foot, the bronchial reflexes between zones 1 and 2 on the ball of the foot, and the diaphragm muscle reflex under the ball of the foot all across zones 1 to 5. Also stimulate the nose and sinus reflexes to help clear any congestion or blockage to free breathing. Working the lung and bronchial reflexes is especially important when there is congestion or asthma.

SEE GOOD STEPS:

For Respiratory Ailments, page 206.

7. THE DIGESTIVE SYSTEM

The digestive system is made up of the mouth, the teeth, the tongue, the salivary glands (chewing starts the process), and esophagus (which relays the food), the stomach and small intestine, where most of the digestive process takes place, and the large intestine, which carries the waste out of the body. The pancreas, liver, and gallbladder aid digestion by releasing digestive enzymes into the small intestine.

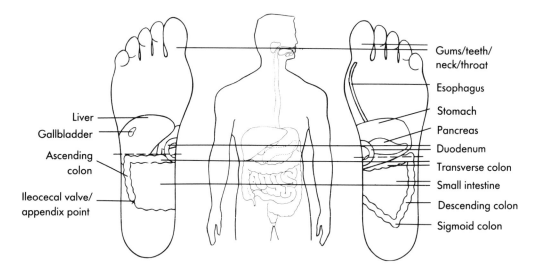

The function of the digestive system is to convert the food we eat into the protein building-blocks of our body and the nutrients needed by every cell for the energy required to maintain life. The digestive system also aids excretion of waste material.

Sometimes the digestive system becomes sluggish. The results of improper digestion and improper elimination are a toxic congestion of the body, tiredness, and lack of vitality and strength.

Therefore, work the entire digestive system, the pancreas, the liver, and the gallbladder on the feet.

SEE GOOD STEPS:

For Indigestion, page 228.

8. THE URINARY SYSTEM

The urinary system is made up of the kidneys, ureters, bladder, and urethra.

Its function is to get rid of urea, a nitrogen waste product resulting from metabolism. Blood is brought to the kidney, where it is filtered to release the urea, other wastes, and substances that are in excess in the blood. Tubules then save valuable water, ions, and glucose for reabsorption. The ureters carry the urine to the bladder for storage, where it is voluntarily released through the urethra.

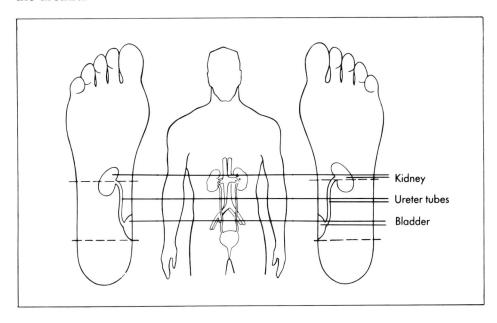

In order to maintain the efficient functioning of the urinary system, we work all the reflexes to this system. This helps to detoxify the body and to prevent or alleviate any blockages or inflammation of this system.

SEE GOOD STEPS:

For Getting Ready for Bed (especially for bedwetters), page 212.
For Bladder Problems, page 233.

9. THE ENDOCRINE SYSTEM

The endocrine system is comprised of all the ductless glands that secrete hormones directly into the blood and regulate the body's functioning. These glands are the pituitary, pineal, thyroid, parathyroids, thymus, adrenals, pancreas, ovaries, and testes. We have discussed the individual function of each of these glands in Chapter Two.

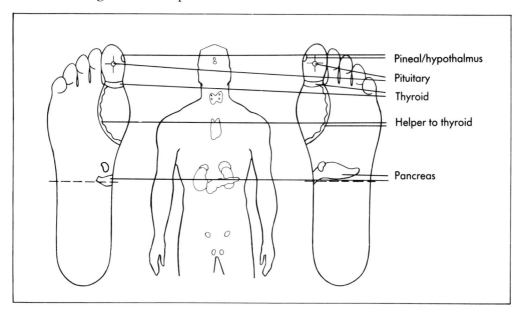

Together, they have a very important role in the body. They regulate the rhythms of life, the emotions, the drives, and when functioning in harmony, they maintain homeostasis, the state of chemical and emotional balance and active health of the body. These reflexes will affect moods, energy, and the proper functioning of all our other systems. So for optimum health and happiness, work the endocrine system on the feet.

SEE GOOD STEPS:

For strengthening endocrine function, work points for all glands above.

10. THE REPRODUCTIVE SYSTEM

The male reproductive system consists of the penis, seminal vesicles, vas deferens, prostate, and testes. In women, the reproductive organs are the vagina, uterus, fallopian tubes, ovaries, and mammary glands.

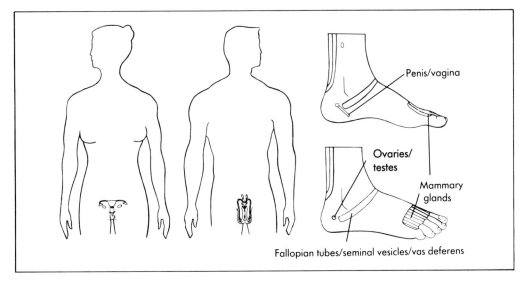

These organs and glands are discussed in Chapter Two. Now let's look at how the full reproductive system affects us.

This system can create new life. In women it maintains and nourishes this new life until birth and feeds it after birth.

This is the process of "generation." There is evidence that the reproductive system produces hormones that also "regenerate" our own bodies. Estrogen in women and testosterone in men are vital to producing the basic protein building-blocks. We still have much to learn about these organs, and the effects of their hormones on the body and on the aging process.

Work the reflex points for the reproductive organs for vitality, energy, and regeneration, as well as to strengthen the organs themselves to help them create and sustain new life.

SEE GOOD STEPS:

For Sexual Dysfunction, page 157.
For Overcoming Infertility, page 182.

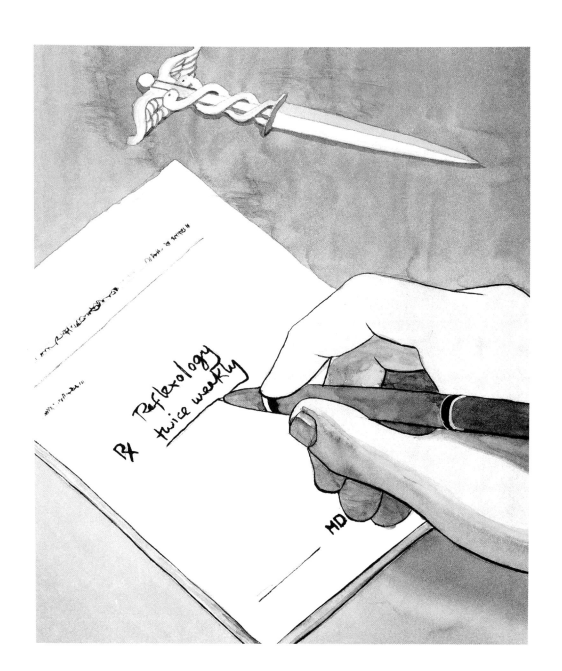

CHAPTER FOURTEEN

REFLEXOLOGY AND THE HEALTH CARE PROFESSIONS

While the purpose of this book is to bring reflexology into the home and workplace, mention should be made about reflexology and the health care professions. I firmly believe that reflexology can improve the health of millions of Americans when given by family members and friends, and that the simple reflexology techniques can be practiced and perfected so that a session at home is as beneficial as one from a professional reflexologist. Yet many people prefer to go to a professional as one of the ways they treat themselves and to keep in touch with the latest developments in the field. Too often they have trouble locating a reflexologist, or their other health care practitioners (physicians, dentists, chiropractors, nutritionists, and psychotherapists) know little about reflexology and cannot advise them.

As more Americans look to holistic methods of staying and being well, it is important for all health care professionals to be approachable and knowledgeable about other fields. In fact, I believe that the trend for the future of health care in America is toward holistic health care centers where a variety of technicians trained in a variety of disciplines are available for the client. Reflexology should be a key service in every health care clinic. Reflexology not only produces a greater sense of well-being when received on a regular basis, but when done immediately before other treatment, such as psychotherapy or dental work, the client/patient relaxes, overcomes fears, and is more open for the healing process to take place.

If you are in one of the health care professions, consider what ways you can make reflexology part of your program. Most professionals do not have the time to learn new techniques or to practice them. A few do. In any event, a reflexologist could be hired as part of the team. In the case of a small clinic, the staff could work in conjunction with an outside reflexologist to whom clients are referred.

Even if you think there is no time for you to add a few minutes of reflexology to your busy practice, I heartily advise your taking a weekend course in it. I think you will find that learning and doing reflexology is not hard or time-consuming. And experiencing it intensively during the classes will introduce you to its wonderful effects. You'll become more knowledgeable about reflexology and be able to speak from experience when your clients or patients ask about it.

Finally, I think that we who promote good health owe it to ourselves to be healthy examples of what we preach. Our clients and patients expect it! Doctors, nurses, dental assistants, hospital staff, and all health care professionals put in long, tiring hours in caring for others. We need to find ways to balance this outpouring of energy and love—ways to receive it back for ourselves. We need to build up and conserve energy and stay calm and centered so that we can bring true peace and healing to the people we serve. Reflexology can be the source of that peace and healing.

CHAPTER FIFTEEN

TABLE OF COMMON CONDITIONS

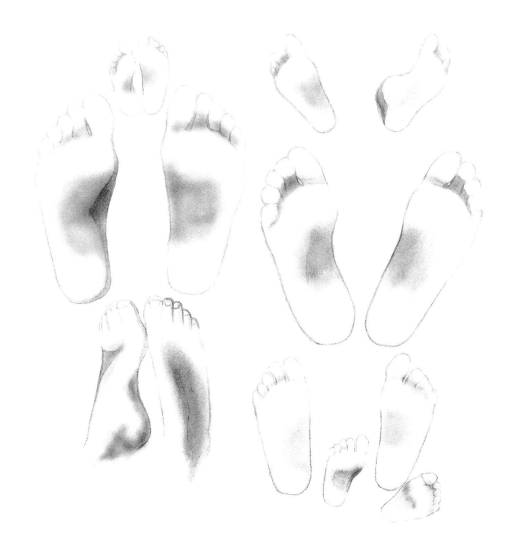

The table is a list of common conditions along with the reflex points on the foot that should be worked to bring relief and healing to the affected area of the body. We have also included an illustration to help you locate the reflex points, and affirmations that will center the mind and emotions on the healing work. Remember that reflexology is not a method of diagnosis. We encourage you to consult a reputable physician for serious problems and to follow the medical advice you receive from him or her. Neither is reflexology meant to replace medication or other therapies prescribed by your family doctor.

AFFIRMATIONS

As mentioned above, the table that follows includes affirmations for each condition. The use of affirmations as a healing tool is based on two beliefs. The first is that at any given moment, we exist on three planes: body, mind, and spirit. An event in one area will have manifestations in the other two. This means, among other things, that an emotional state will have physical ramifications. For instance, anger may manifest physically as an upset stomach, resentment as an ulcer, jealousy as a headache.

The second belief is that the thoughts we have and the words we use define our experiences. How we think of ourselves, our lives, and our relationships in a very real way determines who we are, what our lives are like, how our relationships unfold. The ways in which we mentally and verbally characterize reality limit the reality we experience. And if we change our thought and language patterns, we can change our reality.

These beliefs are not about blaming a person for his or her disorder. Rather they are meant to empower someone who is suffering, to offer the possibility of change to someone who feels victimized.

The affirmations which accompany the list of reflex areas below are based on typical correlations found between emotional states and physical disorders. Each person is unique, however. If an affirmation does not ring true for you, if it doesn't seem to make the statement that you need, please make your own.

CONDITION	DESCRIPTION	REFLEX AREAS	AFFIRMATION
ACNE	Eruptions in the skin	Solar plexus/ diaphragm, chest/ lung, thyroid and helper to thyroid, pituitary, intestines, kidneys, adrenals, liver	My skin is as clear and as pure as my heart.
ADENOID PROBLEMS	Difficulty in breathing due to enlargement of the adenoids	Solar plexus/ diaphragm, chest/ lung, bronchials, sinuses, pituitary	I breathe deeply and fully from the diaphragm.
ALCOHOLISM	Compulsive behavioral pattern leading to abuse of alcoholic substances	Solar plexus/ diaphragm, chest/ lung, bronchials, heart, brain, pineal, pituitary, hypothalamus, pancreas, liver, bladder, ureters, kidneys	I am able to control my life with the help of the Universe. I am able to be the kind of person I truly want to be.

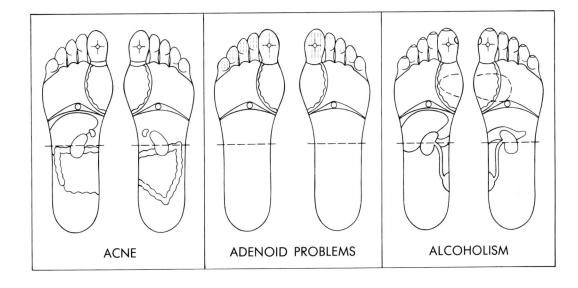

ACNE   ADENOID PROBLEMS   ALCOHOLISM

CONDITION	DESCRIPTION	REFLEX AREAS	AFFIRMATION
ALLERGIES	The body's immune system overreacting to specific foods, materials, pollens, and other substances when in fact there is no danger	a. Solar plexus/ diaphragm, chest/ lung, thyroid and helper to thyroid, all toes with emphasis on pituitary, sinuses ileocecal valve, intestines, adrenals b. Breast/chest, lymph neck/chest, thymus, big toes with emphasis on throat and nose, reproductive glands, chronic reproductive, lymph/groin	I am safe and secure with foods and in my surroundings at all times.
ANEMIA	Iron deficiency in the blood cells	Thyroid and helper to thyroid, heart, spleen, liver	My blood is abundant with life's energy.
ANGINA- PECTORIS	A spasm in the coronary arteries	Solar plexus/ diaphragm, chest/ lung, heart, shoulder/ arm, neck, thoracic and cervical spine, intestines with emphasis on sigmoid colon, duodenum, adrenals	My heart is open to joy and happiness.
APPENDICITIS	Inflammation of the appendix	Solar plexus/ diaphragm, appendix/ileocecal valve, intestines, duodenum, adrenals	I have all the inner peace and tranquility I need.
ARTHRITIS	Inflammation of a joint	Entire foot with emphasis on the following: spine, parathyroids, solar plexus/diaphragm, kidneys, adrenals, reflex for afflicted area	I'm letting go of all the fear, stress, worry, and anxiety I have been holding onto all of my life.

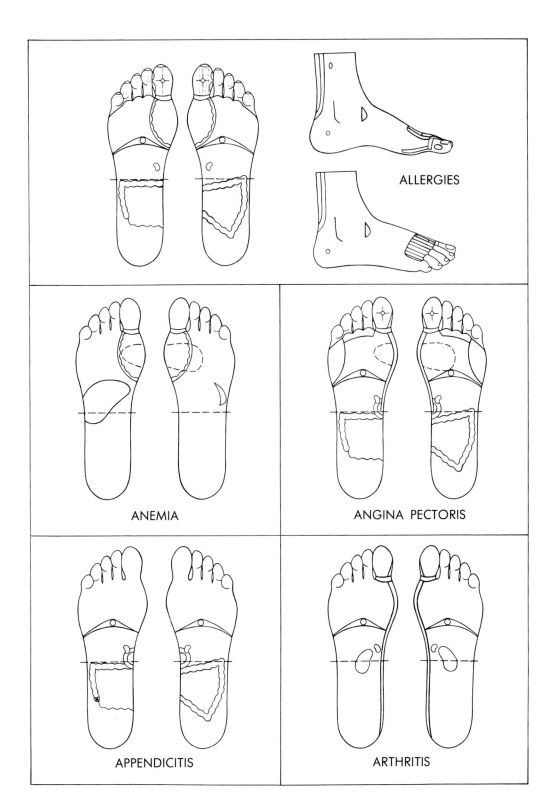

ALLERGIES

ANEMIA

ANGINA PECTORIS

APPENDICITIS

ARTHRITIS

CONDITION	DESCRIPTION	REFLEX AREAS	AFFIRMATION
ASTHMA	Allergic condition expressed through various breathing difficulties such as wheezing and coughing	a. Solar plexus/ diaphragm, chest/ lung, shoulder/arm, bronchials, heart, sinuses, ileocecal valve, intestines, adrenals b. Breast/chest, shoulder/arm, reproductive glands, chronic reproductive	The Universe is providing me with an abundance of breath now and always.
BACK PROBLEMS		a. Solar plexus/ diaphragm, spine, shoulder/arm, neck, sciatic b. Spine, neck, shoulder/arm, mid-back, sciatic, hip/ sciatic	The Universe is backing me up in all my decisions and responsibilities.
(UPPER BACK)		c. Solar plexus/ diaphragm, spine with emphasis on cervical and thoracic spine, shoulder/arm, neck, sciatic	Help and support are always available to me when I need them.
(LOWER BACK)		d. Spine, with emphasis on lumbar, sacral, coccyx, solar plexus/ diaphragm, sciatic Spine, knee/leg/hip, hip/sciatic	My body and my spirit are in perfect alignment with the energies of the Universe.
BEDWETTING		Solar plexus/ diaphragm, spine with emphasis on lumbar, brain, bladder, ureters, kidneys, adrenals	I am in charge of my body and my bed stays dry all night.
BLADDER PROBLEMS	Difficulties in urination	Solar plexus/ diaphragm, chest/ lung, bronchials, lower spine with emphasis on lumbar, bladder, ureters, kidneys, adrenals	I have full control over my bodily functions. I have all the power I need to take charge of my life.

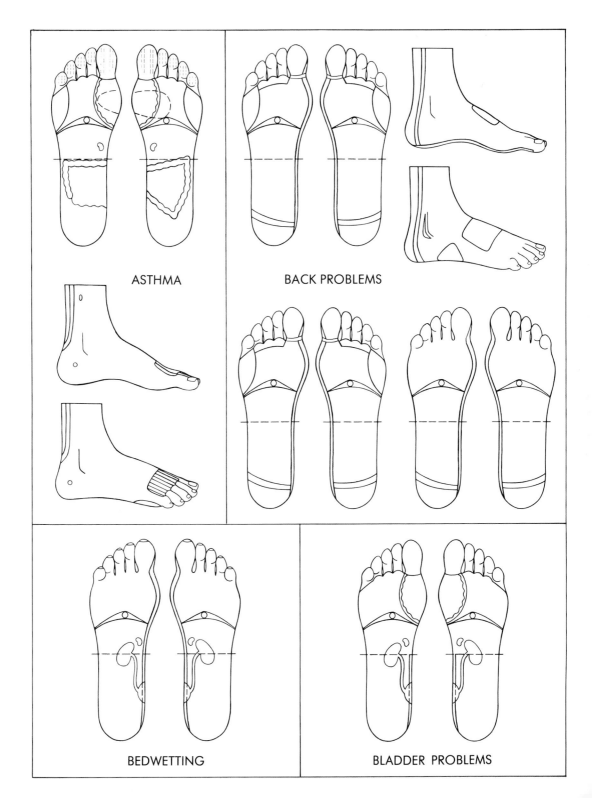

ASTHMA

BACK PROBLEMS

BEDWETTING

BLADDER PROBLEMS

CONDITION	DESCRIPTION	REFLEX AREAS	AFFIRMATION
BREAST (lumps)	Blocked or infected lymph nodes	a. Solar plexus/ diaphragm, chest/ lung, heart, shoulder/ arm, thoracic spine with emphasis on T1–7, pituitary, bladder, ureters, kidneys b. Breast/chest, lymph neck/chest, thymus, mid-back, thoracic spine, bladder	I free myself of all blocked energy. My energy runs as clear as a mountain spring.
BRONCHITIS	Inflammation of the bronchial tubes	a. Solar plexus/ diaphragm, chest/ lung, bronchials, heart, shoulder/arm, thoracic spine with emphasis on T1–7, ileocecal valve, intestines, adrenals b. Breast/chest, lymph neck/chest, shoulder/ arm, thoracic spine, mid-back	With each breath I take I fill myself with love and light. My body nourishes me with more love and light.
BUNIONS (see Calluses)			
BURSITIS	Inflammation of tissue in the joints	a. Solar plexus/ diaphragm, chest/ lung, shoulder/arm, spine, kidneys, adrenals, sciatic, referral area to afflicted part of body b. Breast/chest, lymph neck/chest, shoulder/ arm, spine, mid-back, knee/leg/hip, hip/ sciatic, sciatic, lymph/ groin	I am releasing all the anger and frustration in my life.
CALLUSES	Thickening of outer skin tissue caused by pressure of friction	Work directly on and around the affected area	My life runs smoothly at all times.

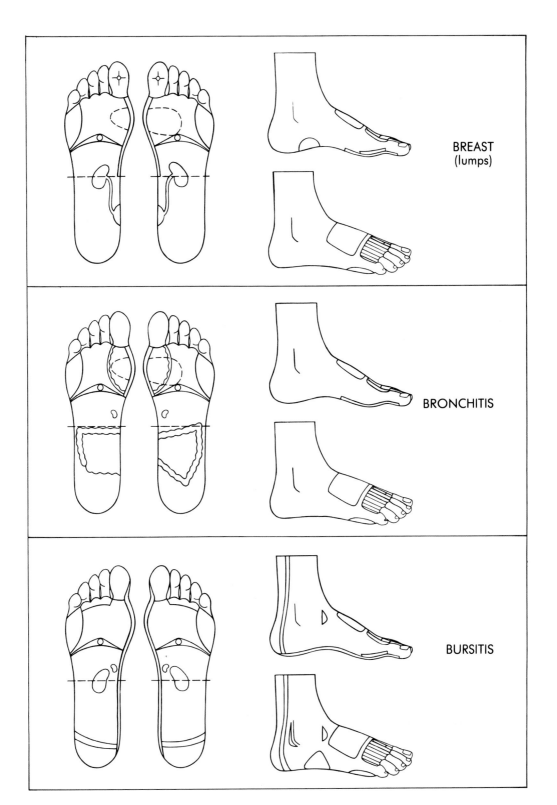

BREAST
(lumps)

BRONCHITIS

BURSITIS

CONDITION	DESCRIPTION	REFLEX AREAS	AFFIRMATION
CATARACTS	Growths over the lens of the eye causing opaque vision	Eye/ear/neck, cervicals, all toes with emphasis on pituitary, thyroid and helper to thyroid, kidneys	I can clearly see all the beauty surrounding me.
CIRRHOSIS OF THE LIVER (see Alcoholism)			
CHOLESTEROL	A sterol synthesized in the liver; implicated in gall stones and arterial plaque	Solar plexus/diaphragm, thyroid and helper to thyroid, heart, liver, gall bladder	I am a clear channel for positive thinking.
COLDS	Various symptoms	a. Solar plexus/diaphragm, chest/lung, bronchials, thyroid and helper to thyroid, shoulder/arm, eye/ear/neck, esophagus, all toes with emphasis on pituitary, stomach, spleen, ileocecal valve, intestines, duodenum, adrenals, liver b. Breast/chest, lymph/neck/chest, inner ear, thymus, shoulder/arm, all toes with emphasis on throat and nose	Nature is cleansing me and I am assisting Her in the process.
COLITIS	Inflammation of the colon	a. Solar plexus/diaphragm, intestines, duodenum, adrenals, liver, gallbladder, lower spine b. Lymph/groin	I can allow myself to experience the happiness and joys of life.
CONJUNCTIVITIS (see Eye Disorders)			

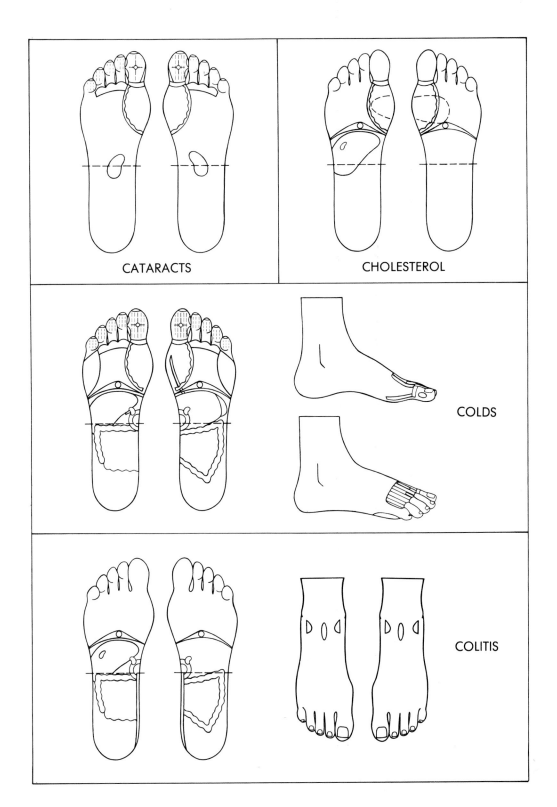

CATARACTS

CHOLESTEROL

COLDS

COLITIS

CONDITION	DESCRIPTION	REFLEX AREAS	AFFIRMATION
CONSTIPATION	Elimination difficulty	a. Solar plexus/ diaphragm, lower spine, spleen, ileocecal valve, intestines, duodenum, adrenals, liver, gallbladder, sciatic b. Lower spine, sciatic, hip/sciatic, hip/knee/ leg	I give myself permission to move ahead with my life.
CORNS (see Calluses)			
CRAMPS	Muscle spasm	a. Solar plexus/ diaphragm, chest/ lung, bronchials, heart, spine, parathyroid, adrenals, sciatic b. Breast/chest, hip/ knee, hip/sciatic, sciatic, spine, mid-back, referral area	I am breathing healing energy into all the muscles of my body.
CRAMPS, MENSTRUAL (see Menstruation)			
CYSTITIS	Bladder inflammation	a. Lower spine, bladder, ureters, kidneys, adrenals b. Lower spine, lymph/ groin, hip/sciatic, hip/ knee, bladder	I am releasing the difficulties and sorrows of my life. My life flows as it must.
DEPRESSION	Emotional lassitude	a. Solar plexus/ diaphragm, chest/ lung, shoulder/arm, neck, heart, thyroid and helper to thyroid, parathyroids, all toes with emphasis on pituitary, brain, pancreas, adrenals b. Breast/chest, thymus, shoulder/arm, neck/ throat	Happiness moves through me like a river of love.
DIABETES	Sugar and insulin disorder in the blood	Solar plexus/ diaphragm, thyroid and helper to thyroid, heart, pituitary, pancreas, liver, adrenals	My blood-sugar level is in perfect harmony and balance.

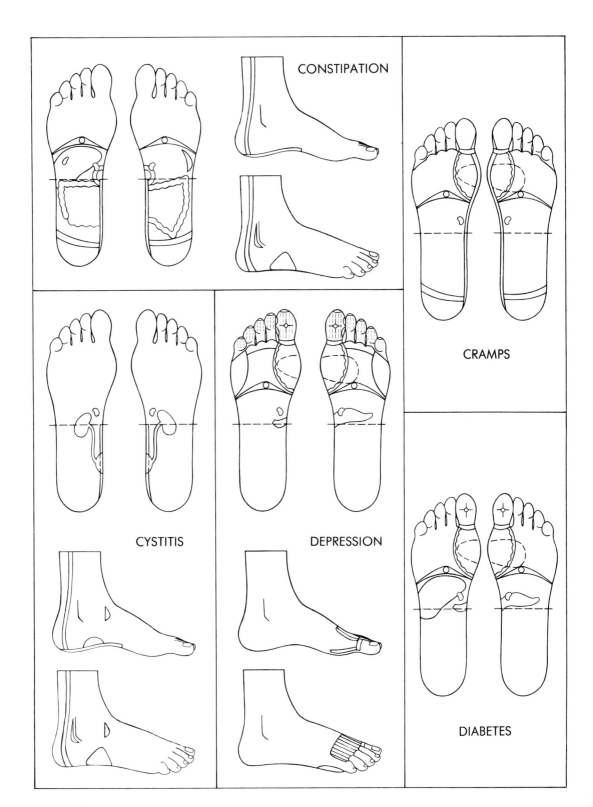

CONSTIPATION

CRAMPS

CYSTITIS

DEPRESSION

DIABETES

CONDITION	DESCRIPTION	REFLEX AREAS	AFFIRMATION
DIARRHEA	Abnormally frequent and fluid bowel movements	a. Solar plexus/ diaphragm, lower spine, ileocecal valve, intestines, duodenum, adrenals, liver b. Lower spine, chronic rectal	I feel grounded, confident, and aware as I go about my everyday life.
DISC PROBLEMS	Pressure resulting from improper alignment of vertebrae	a. Solar plexus/ diaphragm, spine with emphasis on affected area, neck, shoulder/ arm, brain, sciatic b. Spine, neck/throat, shoulder/arm, mid-back, sciatic, hip/ sciatic	I hold my head high and accept life's challenges.
DIVERTICULITIS	Inflammation of the diverticulum sac in the bowel wall	Solar plexus/ diaphragm, lower spine, intestines with emphasis on sigmoid colon, duodenum, adrenals, liver, gallbladder	I surrender the sorrows of the past and make room for the joys of the present.
DIZZINESS	An inner ear condition that causes the physical environment to seem to be spinning	a. Solar plexus/ diaphragm, all toes with emphasis on pituitary, cervicals, helper to eye/ear b. Inner ear, cervicals	My body, mind, and spirit are in perfect balance.
DRUG ADDICTION	Compulsive use of euphoric or depressant substances	a. Solar plexus/ diaphragm, heart, thyroid and helper to thyroid, all toes with emphasis on pituitary and brain, pancreas, liver, kidneys, adrenals, neck b. Thymus, lymph neck/ chest, lymph/groin	I am whole and complete.
DRY SKIN (see Eczema)			

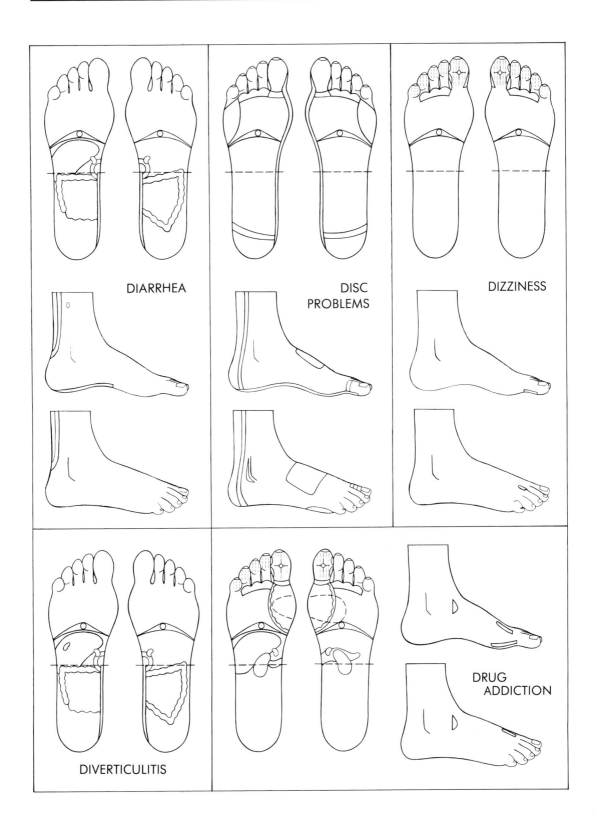

DIARRHEA

DISC
PROBLEMS

DIZZINESS

DIVERTICULITIS

DRUG
ADDICTION

CONDITION	DESCRIPTION	REFLEX AREAS	AFFIRMATION
EARACHE	Infection in the ear	a. Solar plexus/ diaphragm, all toes, cervicals, helper to eye/ear, adrenals b. Thymus, lymph neck/ chest, inner ear, neck/ throat, upper and lower jaw, cervicals	The message and music of life reach my inner ear and I am healed.
ECZEMA	Dryness of the skin	a. Solar plexus/ diaphragm, chest/ lung, thyroid and helper to thyroid, pituitary, intestines, kidneys, duodenum, adrenals, pancreas, liver b. Breast/chest, lymph neck/chest, thymus, lymph/groin	My skin is clear, alive, and glowing. I am in the light.
EDEMA	Swelling due to fluid retention	a. Solar plexus/ diaphragm, heart, bladder, ureters, kidneys, adrenals, reflex and referral for afflicted area b. Lymph neck/chest, lymph/groin, bladder	I feel protected and secure enough to release the excess fluid in my body.
EMPHYSEMA	Inelasticity in lung sac that causes difficulty in breathing	a. Solar plexus/ diaphragm, chest/ lung, bronchials, neck, cervical and thoracic spine, ileocecal valve, intestines, adrenals. b. Breast/chest, lymph neck/chest, throat, nose, cervicals, thoracic spine, mid-back	I am free to be who I want to be.
EPILEPSY	Disorder of the nervous system, typically manifest convulsive attacks	Solar plexus/ diaphragm, spine, neck, throat, thyroid and helper to thyroid, all toes with emphasis on brain and pituitary, pancreas, ileocecal valve, intestines, adrenals	I feel safe and joyous within the eternal flow of life.

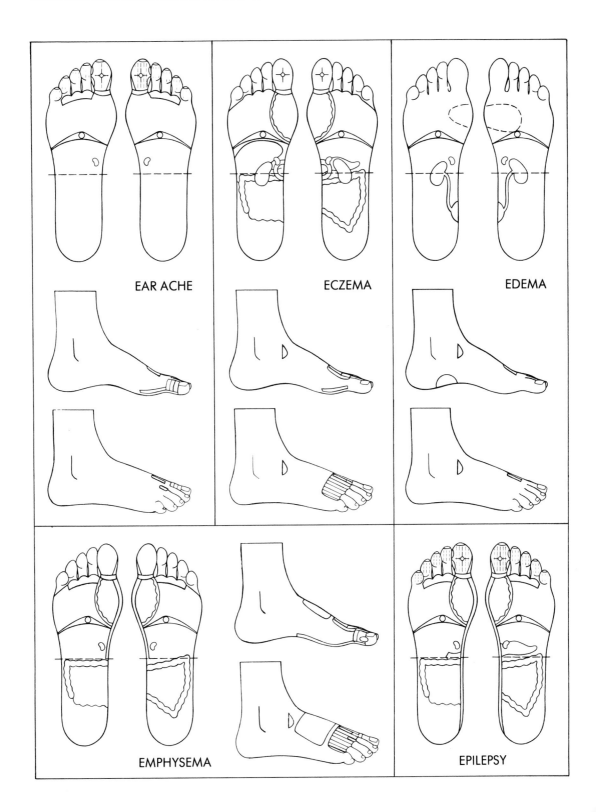

EAR ACHE

ECZEMA

EDEMA

EMPHYSEMA

EPILEPSY

CONDITION	DESCRIPTION	REFLEX AREAS	AFFIRMATION
EYE DISORDERS		Helper to eye/ear, all toes with emphasis on brain, cervicals, kidneys	I can now see exactly what I need to see around me to feel completely fulfilled.
FAINTING	Loss of consciousness by insufficient blood to the brain	Heart, all toes with emphasis on pituitary and brain, cervicals	Choices, commitments, and lessons are easy for me to handle.
FATIGUE	Weariness or exhaustion from overexertion	Solar plexus/ diaphragm, heart, thyroid and helper to thyroid, spine, all toes with emphasis on pituitary and brain, spleen, pancreas, liver, adrenals	I am alive, alert, and refreshed.
FEVER	Increased body temperature associated with infection and other illnesses	a. Thyroid and helper to thyroid, all toes with emphasis on brain, pituitary and hypothalamus, cervicals, kidneys, spleen, uterus, bladder, and liver b. Lymph, neck/chest, thymus, cervicals, lymph/groin	I express my love for life coolly and calmly.
FLATULENCE	Excessive gas in stomach or intestines	Solar plexus/ diaphragm, esophagus, lower spine, intestines with emphasis on sigmoid colon, duodenum, stomach, pancreas, liver, gallbladder	I assimilate my life and digest my food with great ease and comfort.
FRACTURE	Broken bones tissue	Corresponding part of foot referral areas	My life is whole. I grow stronger every day.

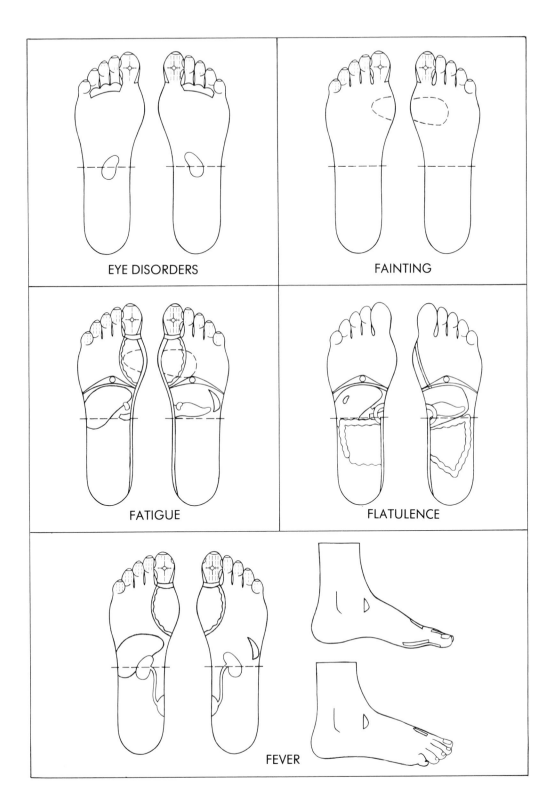

EYE DISORDERS

FAINTING

FATIGUE

FLATULENCE

FEVER

CONDITION	DESCRIPTION	REFLEX AREAS	AFFIRMATION
GALLSTONES	Crystallized fatty congestions, especially cholesterol	Solar plexus/ diaphragm, thyroid and helper to thyroid, thoracic spine, liver, gallbladder	I replace negative thoughts and harshness with love and laughter.
GAS PAINS (see Flatulence)			
GLAUCOMA	Increased pressure caused by excess fluid in the eyeball	Solar plexus/ diaphragm, helper to eye/ear, all toes with emphasis on pituitary, cervicals, kidneys	I see all the good things about life and I rejoice in them.
GOUT	Inflamed joint caused by excess uric acid in blood	a. Solar plexus/ diaphragm, liver, kidneys, referral and reflex for afflicted area b. Lymph neck/chest, lymph/groin	I am patient and I feel safe with others. I have no need to dominate.
GROWTHS, ABNORMAL		Referral and reflex for afflicted area, pituitary, spleen	I forgive all the people in life I feel have wronged me. I let go of all the situations that feel unfair. I praise what I have done well and fill myself with the ease of loving myself.
HALITOSIS	Bad breath	a. Solar plexus/ diaphragm, esophagus, stomach, duodenum, liver, intestines, all toes b. Teeth, gums/upper jaw, teeth, gums/ lower jaw	I breathe in healing energy and exhale the refreshing sweetness of life.

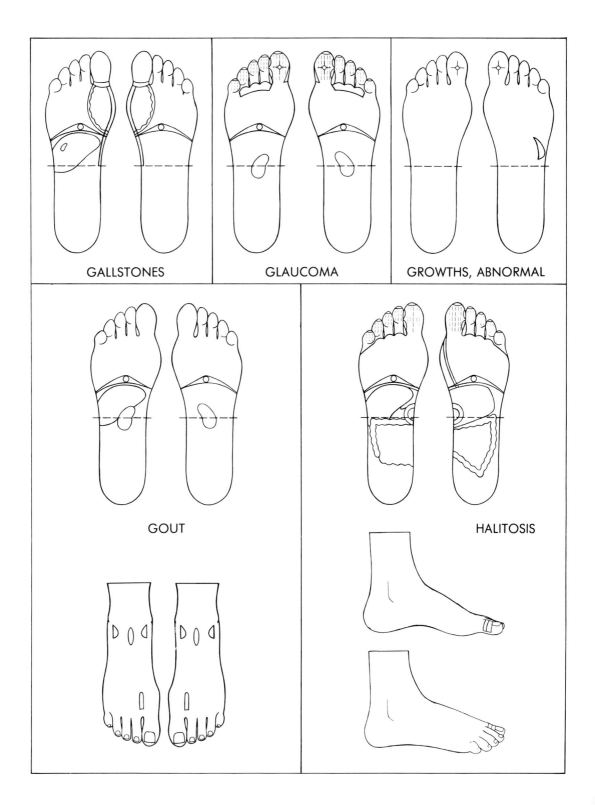

GALLSTONES

GLAUCOMA

GROWTHS, ABNORMAL

GOUT

HALITOSIS

CONDITION	DESCRIPTION	REFLEX AREAS	AFFIRMATION
HAY FEVER	Allergic reaction to pollen	a. Solar plexus/ diaphragm, chest/ lung, bronchials, cervicals, neck, all toes with emphasis on sinuses and pituitary, eyes, ileocecal valve, intestines, adrenals b. Breast/chest, lymph neck/chest, thymus, throat/neck and nose, cervicals, lymph/ groin, reproductive glands, chronic reproductive	I am letting go of all my guilty feelings as I walk peacefully through a safe and friendly world.
HEADACHE		a. Solar plexus/ diaphragm, shoulder/ arm, neck, thyroid and helper to thyroid, spine with emphasis on cervicals, all toes with emphasis on pituitary, brain and sinuses, pancreas, ileocecal valve, intestines, adrenals, sciatic b. Spine, thymus, lymph neck/chest, neck/ throat, upper and lower jaw, mid-back, reproductive glands, chronic reproductive, sciatic, hip/sciatic, breast/chest and shoulder/arm	I resolve all conflicts easily and effortlessly.
HEARING PROBLEMS		Shoulder/arm, eye/ear/ neck, all toes with emphasis on brain, pituitary and sinuses, cervicals	I am listening to the harmonies of the Universe.

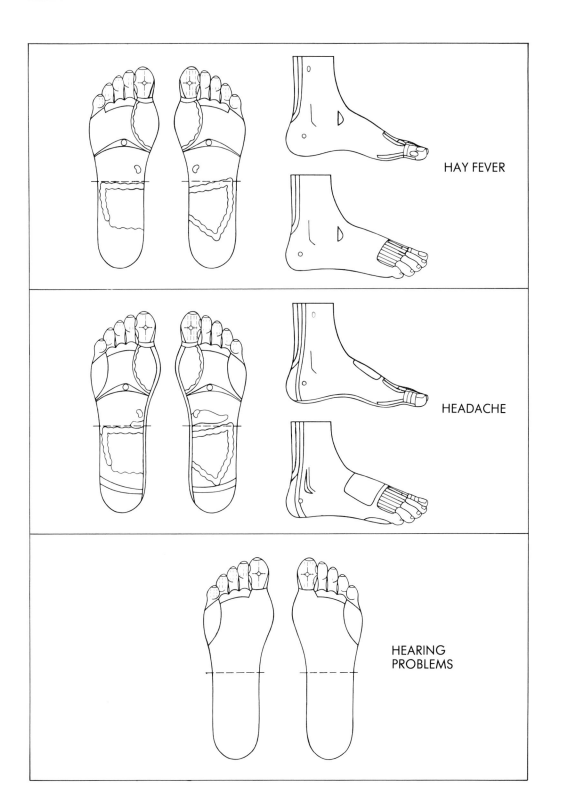

HAY FEVER

HEADACHE

HEARING
PROBLEMS

CONDITION	DESCRIPTION	REFLEX AREAS	AFFIRMATION
HEART ATTACK	Insufficient blood through a coronary artery blocked by blood clot or plaque	Solar plexus/ diaphragm, chest/ lung, heart, shoulder/ arm, spine with emphasis on thoracic spine, brain, pituitary, intestines with emphasis on sigmoid, colon, kidneys, adrenals	My heart is filled with unconditional love.
HEARTBURN	A burning sensation in the stomach, often extending to the esophagus	Solar plexus/ diaphragm, chest/ lung, heart, esophagus, thoracic spine, intestines, duodenum, pancreas, stomach, gallbladder	I breathe fully, trusting life and releasing fear.
HEMORRHOIDS	Varicose veins in the rectum	a. Solar plexus/ diaphragm, heart, lumbar, coccyx, sacral, intestines with emphasis on sigmoid colon, adrenals, sciatic b. Sciatic, chronic rectum, hip/sciatic, hip/knee/leg, lower spine	I have time and energy to do everything I need to do.
HERNIA	Protrusion of an organ through the wall of the cavity that contains it	a. Solar plexus/ diaphragm, lower spine, intestines, adrenals b. Lower spine, hip, hip/ sciatic, knee, lymph/ groin	I am relieved of the pressures and burdens of the day.
HIATAL HERNIA	Protrusion of the stomach through the diaphragm	Solar plexus/ diaphragm, chest/ lung, esophagus, thoracic spine, stomach, adrenals	My mind fills with gentle, harmonious thoughts.
HICCOUGHS	Uncontrollable spasmodic coughing caused by involuntary contractions of the diaphragm	Solar plexus/ diaphragm, chest/ lung, heart, esophagus, bronchials, shoulder/ arm, thoracic spine, neck, toes, stomach	I am releasing fear and speaking freely.

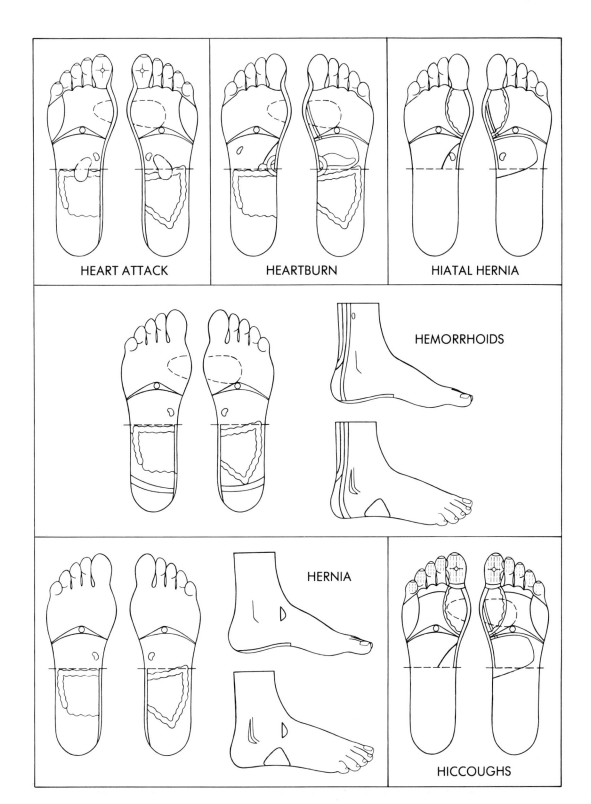

HEART ATTACK

HEARTBURN

HIATAL HERNIA

HEMORRHOIDS

HERNIA

HICCOUGHS

CONDITION	DESCRIPTION	REFLEX AREAS	AFFIRMATION
HIGH BLOOD PRESSURE (also Hypertension)	Condition in which the heart must pump under excessive pressure	Solar plexus/ diaphragm, chest/ lung, spine, heart, thyroid, and helper to thyroid, pituitary, kidneys, adrenals	I allow joy to flow through my entire body freely and easily.
HIP PROBLEMS		a. Solar plexus/ diaphragm, shoulder, lower back with emphasis on sacral, sciatic b. Lower back, sciatic, hip/sciatic, hip/knee, shoulder, lymph groin	I trust in the process of life and move toward my future with happiness and confidence.
HOT FLASHES (see Menopause)			
HYPERACTIVITY	Increased or excessive activity	Solar plexus/ diaphragm, thyroid and helper to thyroid, brain, pituitary, adrenals, pancreas, liver	I am slowing down to move gently through life with enjoyment.
HYPOGLYCEMIA	Deficiency of blood sugar	Thyroid and helper to thyroid, pituitary, pancreas, liver, kidneys, adrenals	My life is in perfect harmony with my highest aspirations.
HYSTERECTOMY	Removal of the uterus	a. Solar plexus/ diaphragm, thyroid and helper to thyroid, pituitary, lower back, sciatic, adrenals b. Chronic reproductive, lower back, sciatic, hip/sciatic, reproductive glands, fallopian tubes, lymph/groin, hip/ knee, thymus	Each day I bless my womanhood and find serenity in Mother Earth.

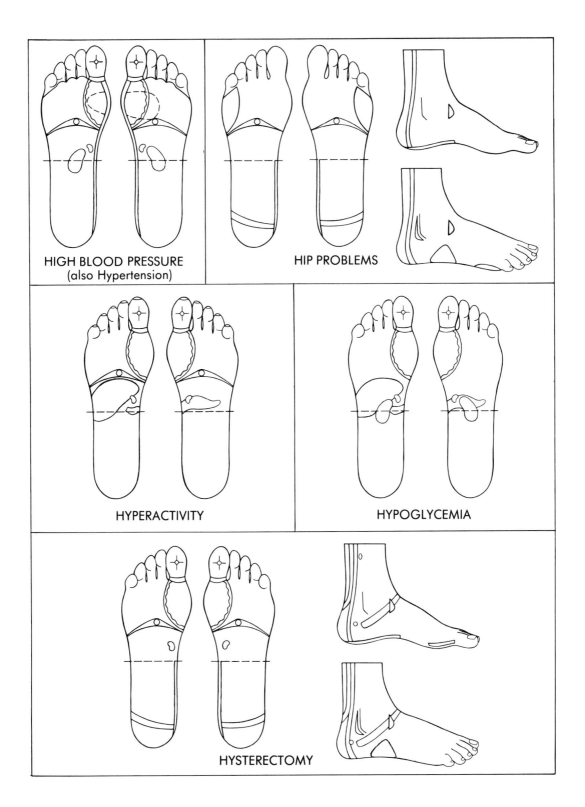

HIGH BLOOD PRESSURE
(also Hypertension)

HIP PROBLEMS

HYPERACTIVITY

HYPOGLYCEMIA

HYSTERECTOMY

CONDITION	DESCRIPTION	REFLEX AREAS	AFFIRMATION
IMPOTENCE	Failure to get or maintain an erection	a. Solar plexus/ diaphragm, chest/ lung, thyroid and helper to thyroid, brain, pituitary, lower spine, pancreas and adrenals b. Breast/chest, thymus, lower back, chronic reproductive, reproductive glands, penis, seminal vesicles, hip/sciatic, hip/knee	I am stimulated by the sensuality of my surroundings and express it in an appropriate, creative fashion.
INCONTINENCE	Inability to control urination	Solar plexus/ diaphragm, lower back, bladder, ureters, kidneys, adrenals	My life is a gift and I have the ability to create it anew each day.
INDIGESTION	Faulty digestive functioning	a. Solar plexus/ diaphragm, thoracic and lumbar spine, esophagus, stomach, pancreas, liver, gallbladder, duodenum, intestines b. Gums, teeth, neck/ throat, lower spine	The Universe feeds my soul with supportive and harmonious experiences.
INFECTIONS	Condition caused by the invasion of bacteria into the body	a. Adrenals, tonsils, thymus, spleen b. Thymus, lymph neck/ chest, lymph/groin Reflex to afflicted area	I easily turn life's little annoyances into life's loving lessons.
INFERTILITY	Inability to conceive a child	a. Solar plexus/ diaphragm, thyroid and helper to thyroid, brain, pituitary, lower back, adrenals b. Chronic reproductive, reproductive glands, fallopian tubes/ seminal vesicles, lower back	I easily flow with the life energies of the Universe.

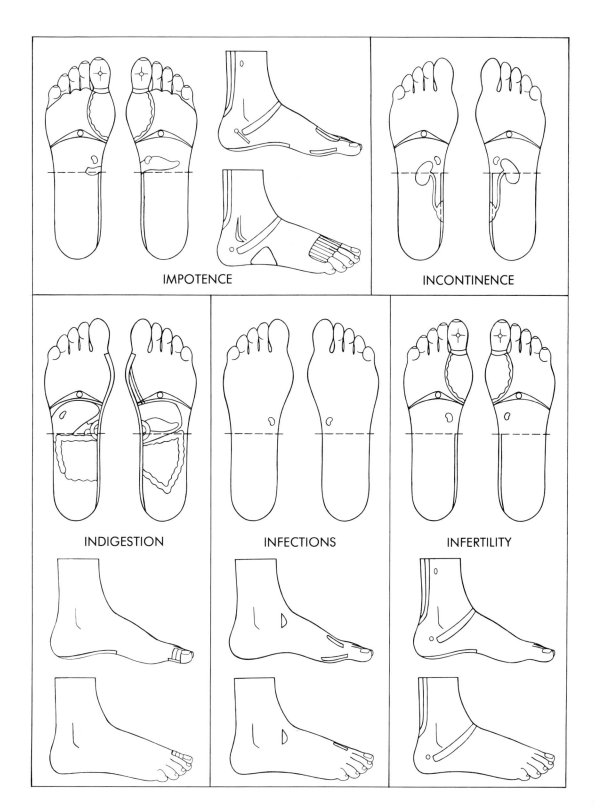

IMPOTENCE

INCONTINENCE

INDIGESTION

INFECTIONS

INFERTILITY

CONDITION	DESCRIPTION	REFLEX AREAS	AFFIRMATION
INFLUENZA	Viral disease characterized by fever, prostration, aches and pains, and inflammation of the respiratory system	a. Solar plexus/diaphragm, chest/lung, bronchials, thyroid and helper to thyroid, all toes with emphasis on pituitary, intestines, adrenals b. Breast/chest, lymph neck/chest, thymus, lymph/groin	With each breath I take, I am confronted by a friendly Universe.
INSOMNIA	Inability to sleep	Solar plexus/diaphragm, chest/lung, shoulder, neck, thyroid and helper to thyroid, all toes with emphasis on brain, pineal and pituitary, pancreas, adrenals	A kind and forgiving world sings me to a peaceful sleep.
JAUNDICE	A yellow condition of the skin due to bile disorder	Thoracic spine, liver, gallbladder	Compassion touches my soul and my soul reflects back the multicolored rainbow of tolerance.
KIDNEY PROBLEMS	Inability to filter; blockage of urine flow	Solar plexus/diaphragm, lower back, bladder, ureters, kidneys, adrenals	I love who I am. All things work for my highest good.
KIDNEY STONES	Crystallizations in the urine	Solar plexus/diaphragm, parathyroid, lower back, bladder, ureters, kidneys, adrenals	All I need to be is crystal clear to me.
KNEE PROBLEMS		a. Spine, shoulder, sciatic; referral area is elbow b. Spine, sciatic, hip/sciatic, knee/leg/hip, mid-back, shoulder	Like a tree in the breeze, I bend with the will of the Universe.

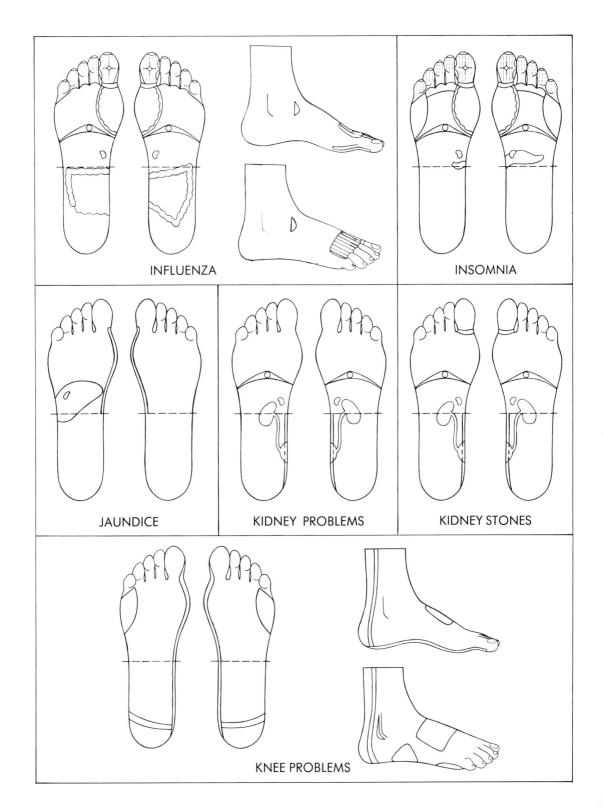

INFLUENZA

INSOMNIA

JAUNDICE

KIDNEY PROBLEMS

KIDNEY STONES

KNEE PROBLEMS

CONDITION	DESCRIPTION	REFLEX AREAS	AFFIRMATION
LARYNGITIS	Inflammation of the larynx	a. Solar plexus/ diaphragm, chest/ lung, neck, all toes cervicals, adrenals b. Breast/chest, lymph neck/chest, vocal cords, neck/throat	All I need to say is "I love you."
LEG PROBLEMS		a. Spine, shoulder, kidneys, adrenals, sciatic, referral for afflicted area b. Spine, sciatic, hip/ sciatic, knee/leg/hip, lymph/groin, mid-back, shoulder	I release the past and move forward into a bright future.
LIVER CONDITIONS		Solar plexus/ diaphragm, chest/ lung, heart, thoracic spine, liver, gallbladder	I am open and receptive to the love in my heart.
LOW BLOOD PRESSURE (also Hypotension)		Solar plexus/ diaphragm, chest/ lung, heart, thyroid and helper to thyroid, parathyroids, pituitary, kidneys, adrenals	I rise to new heights of joyousness and acceptance.
MENOPAUSE	Hot flashes and emotional upsets caused by cessation of menses	a. Solar plexus/ diaphragm, thyroid and helper to thyroid, parathyroids, brain, pituitary, kidneys, adrenals b. Chronic reproductive, reproductive glands, fallopian tube, hip/ sciatic, hip/knee	I am only just beginning a life of comfort, acceptance, and self love.

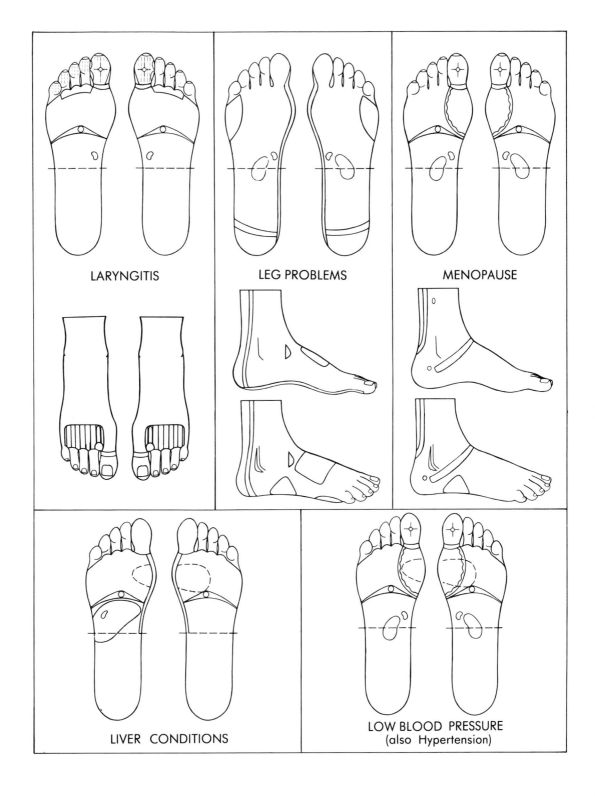

LARYNGITIS

LEG PROBLEMS

MENOPAUSE

LIVER CONDITIONS

LOW BLOOD PRESSURE
(also Hypertension)

CONDITION	DESCRIPTION	REFLEX AREAS	AFFIRMATION
MENSTRUATION	Cramps, irritability, fatigue during menstrual period	a. Solar plexus/diaphragm, chest/lung, thyroid and helper to thyroid, parathyroids, brain, pituitary, pancreas, adrenals, lower back b. Breast/chest, lymph neck/chest, thymus, lower back, chronic reproductive, reproductive glands, hip/sciatic, hip/knee, lymph/groin	I am one with the Universe. My bodily functions are beautifully ordered.
MIGRAINE (see Headache)			
MORNING SICKNESS	Nausea that occurs during first months of pregnancy	a. Solar plexus/diaphragm, thyroid and helper to thyroid, pituitary, stomach, adrenals b. Chronic reproductive, reproductive glands	I awake joyfully to the new life within me.
MOTION SICKNESS	Nausea induced by motion	a. Solar plexus/diaphragm, spine, helper to eye/ear, brain, pituitary, stomach b. Spine, inner ear, mid-back	I travel on a path of least resistance.
NAUSEA	Stomach distress that induces vomiting	Solar plexus/diaphragm, chest/lung, thyroid and helper to thyroid, esophagus, pituitary, stomach, liver, gallbladder, adrenals	I trust in the safety of my life. All is well.
NECK PROBLEMS	Physical injuries or tension	Solar plexus/diaphragm, shoulder, neck, spine, with emphasis on cervicals, all toes, adrenals	I am flexible. I turn to see the beauty in my life.

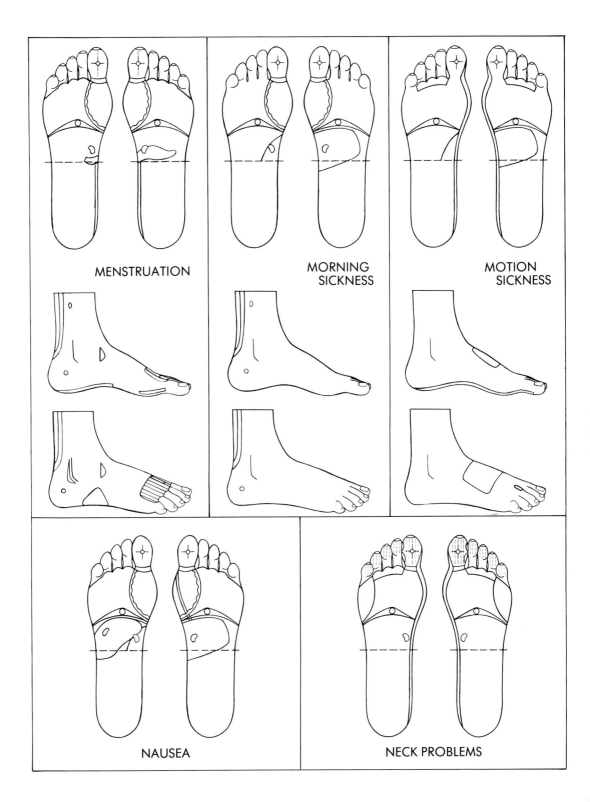

MENSTRUATION

MORNING
SICKNESS

MOTION
SICKNESS

NAUSEA

NECK PROBLEMS

CONDITION	DESCRIPTION	REFLEX AREAS	AFFIRMATION
NERVOUSNESS		Solar plexus/ diaphragm, thyroid and helper to thyroid, spine, brain, pituitary, adrenals, pancreas	I have time to feel the peace, comfort, and joy that is in my life.
NUMBNESS IN FINGERTIPS		Solar plexus/ diaphragm, shoulder/ arm, heart, spine with emphasis on seventh cervical; referral area is all toes	I am open and responsive to the light of the Universe.
PARALYSIS	Complete or partial loss of ability to move or sense with some part of the body	Entire foot with emphasis on solar plexus/diaphragm, spine, neck and brain, reflex for afflicted area	I am at peace inside my body.
PERSPIRING HANDS/FEET		Solar plexus/ diaphragm, thyroid and helper to thyroid, pituitary, liver, intestines, kidneys, adrenals	I remain cool and calm under any adversity.
PHLEBITIS	Inflammation of the wall of a vein	a. Solar plexus/ diaphragm, heart, liver, intestines, adrenals, sciatic; referral area is arm b. Sciatic, hip/sciatic, knee/leg/hip, lymph/ groin, thymus	I create all the joy and happiness I need. My life's energy is unlimited.
PNEUMONIA	Inflammation of the lungs due to bacteria and viruses	a. Solar plexus/ diaphragm, chest/ lung, shoulder/arm, neck, thyroid and helper to thyroid, thoracic spine, intestines, adrenals, pituitary b. Breast/chest, shoulder/arm, lymph neck/chest, thymus, thoracic spine, neck/ throat	My breath expands to the richness around me. I have a new way of looking at life.

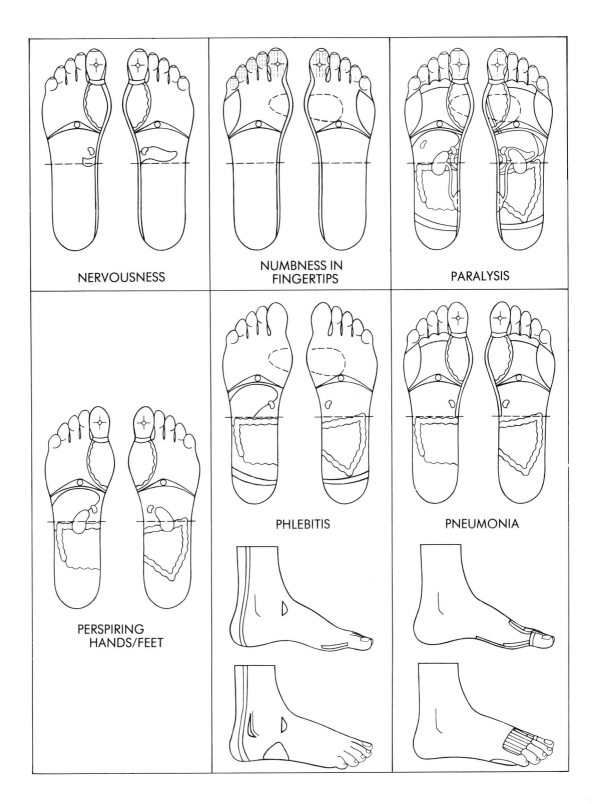

NERVOUSNESS

NUMBNESS IN
FINGERTIPS

PARALYSIS

PERSPIRING
HANDS/FEET

PHLEBITIS

PNEUMONIA

CONDITION	DESCRIPTION	REFLEX AREAS	AFFIRMATION
PREGNANCY		a. Solar plexus/ diaphragm, thyroid and helper to thyroid, spine, pituitary, sciatic, bladder, adrenals b. Breast/chest, thymus, lymph neck/chest, mid-back, spine, sciatic, chronic reproductive, reproductive glands, vagina, fallopian tubes, hip/sciatic, knee/leg/hip, bladder	I rejoice and give thanks for the new life within me.
PROSTATE PROBLEMS	Usually an enlarged prostate gland causing discomfort while urinating	a. Solar plexus/ diaphragm, pituitary, lower back, bladder, adrenals, sciatic b. Lower back, sciatic, chronic reproductive, reproductive glands, seminal vesicles, lymph/groin, bladder	Vital life-force energy flows through me easily and effortlessly.
PSORIASIS	A skin disorder characterized by thickened, red or silver patches	Solar plexus/ diaphragm, chest/ lung, thyroid and helper to thyroid, pituitary, intestines, kidneys, adrenals, liver	I take pleasure in the full acceptance of my life.
RHEUMATISM (see Arthritis and Bursitis)			
SCIATICA	Chronic pain along the sciatic nerve	a. Solar plexus/ diaphragm, shoulder, spine, sciatic b. Shoulder/arm, sciatic, hip/sciatic, knee/leg/ hip, lymph/groin, spine, mid-back	I am safe to move in new directions.

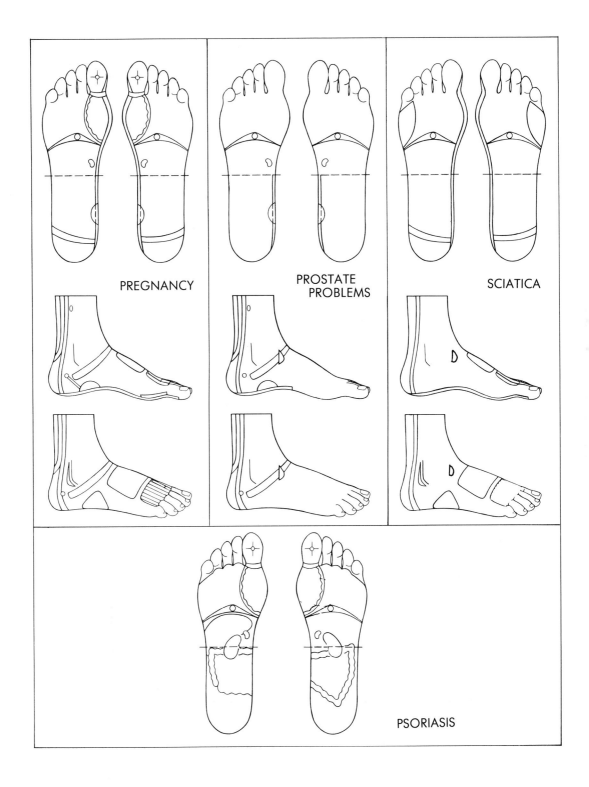

PREGNANCY

PROSTATE PROBLEMS

SCIATICA

PSORIASIS

CONDITION	DESCRIPTION	REFLEX AREAS	AFFIRMATION
SCOLIOSIS	Lateral curvature of the spine; sometimes accompanied by round shoulders or swayback	Solar plexus/ diaphragm, chest/ lung, shoulder/arm, neck, thyroid and helper to thyroid, spine, pituitary, adrenals	I reach for the sky and stretch beyond my limits.
SHINGLES	A virus producing pain and eruptions along the sensory nerves that are afflicted usually in the chest area	a. Solar plexus/ diaphragm, chest/ lung, shoulder/arm, neck, thyroid and helper to thyroid, spine, pituitary, adrenals b. Breast/chest, lymph neck/chest, shoulder/ arm, thymus, neck/ throat, spine, lymph/ groin	I am relaxing and trusting in the healing process.
SHOULDER PAINS		a. Solar plexus/ diaphragm, chest/ lung, shoulder/arm, neck, spine with emphasis on upper back b. Breast/chest, lymph neck/chest, shoulder/ arm, mid-back, hip/ sciatic, hip/knee, spine	I carry my responsibilities with grace and dignity.
SINUSITIS	Congested or clogged sinus cavities	Solar plexus/ diaphragm, chest/ lung, bronchials, neck, all toes with emphasis on sinuses and pituitary, cervicals, ileocecal valve, intestines, adrenals	I can breathe freely because I am free.
SKIN DISORDERS		a. Solar plexus/ diaphragm, thyroid and helper to thyroid, pituitary, intestines, kidneys, adrenals b. Reproductive glands	I am free of past fears and anxieties. I live fully in the moment.

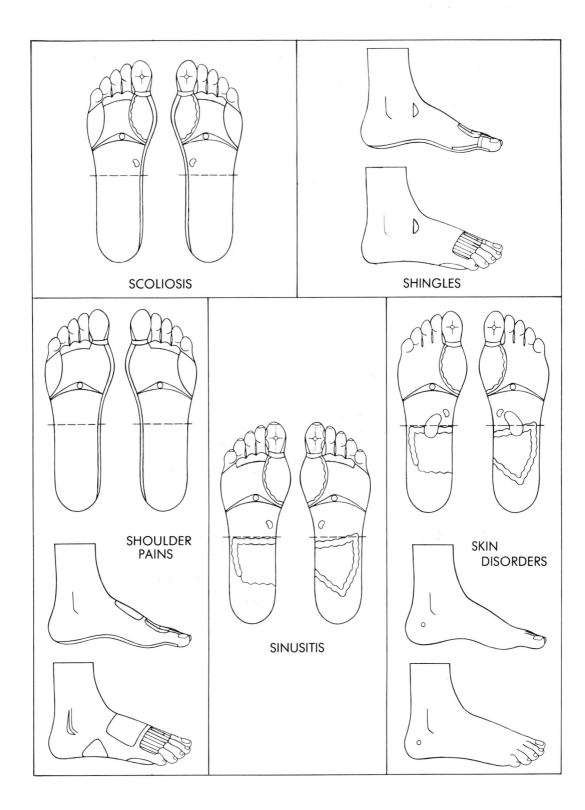

SCOLIOSIS

SHINGLES

SHOULDER PAINS

SINUSITIS

SKIN DISORDERS

CONDITION	DESCRIPTION	REFLEX AREAS	AFFIRMATION
SORE THROAT	Any throat irritation resulting from viral or bacterial infection or from physical stress	a. Solar plexus/ diaphragm, neck, all toes, cervicals, adrenals b. Lymph neck/chest, thymus, cervicals, neck/throat	I express my feelings openly and comfortably.
SPRAIN	Strained, stretched or torn ligaments in a joint	a. Solar plexus/ diaphragm, chest/ lung, heart, adrenals, reflex for afflicted area b. Breast/chest, lymph neck/chest, lymph/ groin	I grow stronger and let the healing energy flow through me.
SPUR ON HEEL	Mineral buildup on a bone in the heel area		I am free to move as I please. Nothing stands in my way.
STROKE	A rupture or blood clot in a vessel of the brain	Solar plexus/ diaphragm, heart, spine, all toes with emphasis on brain (opposite side from the paralysis), reflex for afflicted area	I accept the changes in my life and look forward to what is new.
TEETH AND GUM DISORDERS		a. All toes, cervicals b. Lymph neck/chest, neck/throat, teeth/ gums upper jaw, teeth/gums lower jaw	My teeth and gums are strong, attractive, and serve me well.
TINNITUS	Buzzing, ringing, or hissing in the ear	Solar plexus/ diaphragm, eye/ear/ neck, all toes, cervicals, adrenals	I am able to accept the inner workings of my mind in peace and harmony.

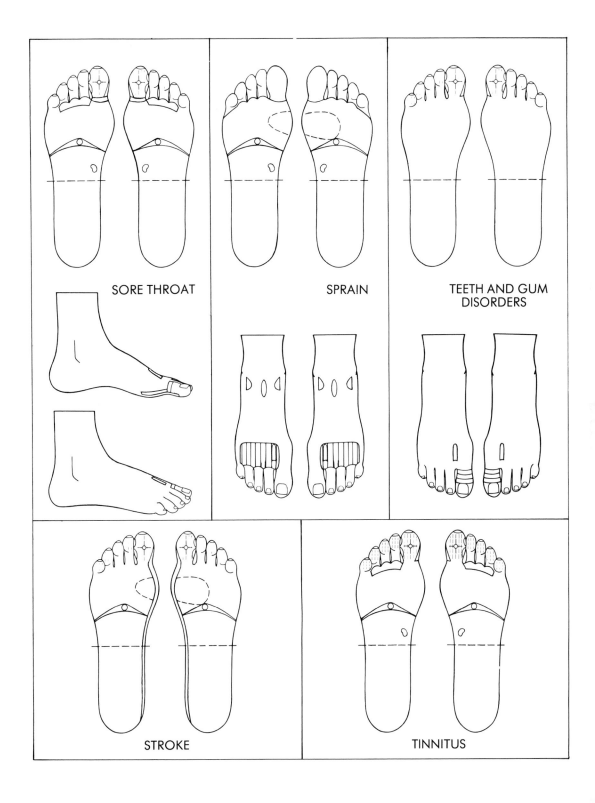

SORE THROAT

SPRAIN

TEETH AND GUM
DISORDERS

STROKE

TINNITUS

CONDITION	DESCRIPTION	REFLEX AREAS	AFFIRMATION
TONSILLITIS	Infection of the tonsils	a. Solar plexus/ diaphragm, eye/ear/ neck, all toes, cervicals, adrenals b. Lymph neck/chest, thymus, cervicals, neck/throat	I am communicating freely, clearly, and honestly.
TUMORS	Growth or enlargement of tissue	Thyroid and helper to thyroid, pituitary, adrenals, reflex for afflicted area	I am releasing the old and welcoming the new.
ULCER	A break in the skin or a mucous membrane that fails to heal	a. Solar plexus/ diaphragm, chest/ lung, heart, esophagus, thyroid and helper to thyroid, neck, thoracic and lumbar spine, stomach, intestines, duodenum, adrenals b. Breast/chest, lymph neck/chest, thymus, thoracic and lumbar spine, lymph/groin, mid-back	All my abilities, strengths, and powers are abundant and free-flowing.
VARICOSE VEINS	Bluish veins	Solar plexus/ diaphragm, chest/ lung, heart, thyroid and helper to thyroid, pituitary, liver, intestines, adrenals, reflex for afflicted area	I move freely through life and enjoy what it offers.
VERTIGO (see Dizziness)			
VITALITY LOSS		Solar plexus/ diaphragm, thyroid and helper to thyroid, spine, brain, pituitary, adrenals, pancreas	I have new energy and enthusiasm.

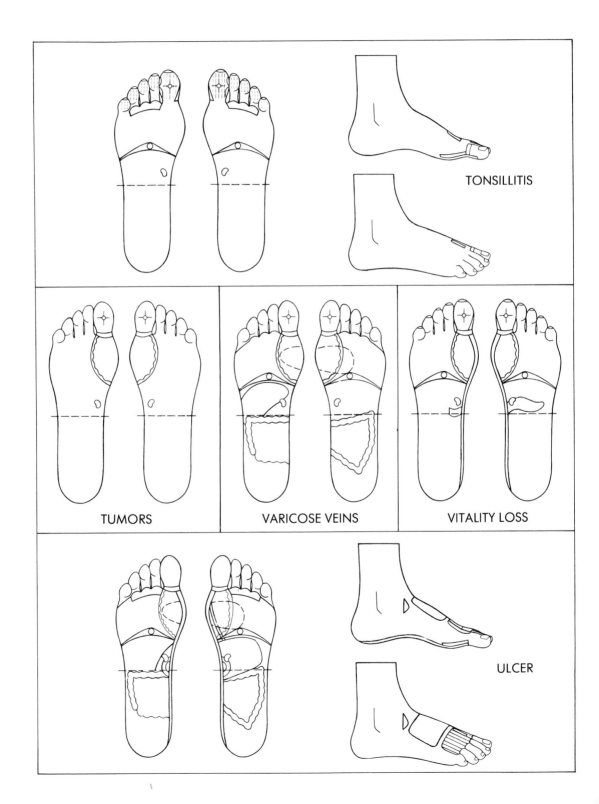

TONSILLITIS

TUMORS

VARICOSE VEINS

VITALITY LOSS

ULCER

CONDITION	DESCRIPTION	REFLEX AREAS	AFFIRMATION
WHIPLASH	Injury to the muscles and tendons in the back of the neck	a. Solar plexus/ diaphragm, chest/ lung, shoulder/arm, neck, spine with emphasis on cervicals, adrenals b. Breast/chest, lymph neck/chest, neck/ throat, shoulder, spine, mid-back	I allow healing energy to flow through my neck and back. I stand straight and tall.

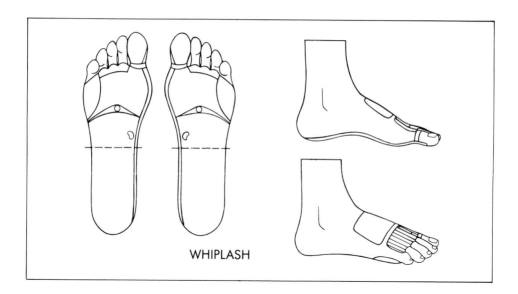

WHIPLASH

INDEX

aches, sedentary, 137–38
Achilles tendon area, 90
Achilles tendon stretch, 59, 108
acne, 171–72, 216, 287
addictive behavior, 255–66
    alcohol and drug abuse, 216, 256,
        257–59, 265, 266, 287, 298,
        299
    buddy system and, 264
    overcoming, 256–57, 264–65
    reflexology in overcoming of, 265–
        266
    smoking, 259–61
    weight loss and, 261–63
adenoids, 276, 287
adrenals, 23, 36, 130, 222, 243, 280
    specific advice for, 83, 116, 118
affirmations, 286
aging, 220
AIDS, 267–68
alcohol, before sessions, 95, 102
alcohol abuse, 216, 256, 257–59, 265,
    266, 287
allergies, 206–7, 288, 290
alpha state, 163
alternating thumb rotations, 53, 107,
    110
anemia, 276, 288, 289
angina-pectoris, 288, 289
ankle area, 41–43, 92–93
ankle boogie, 56, 108
ankle rocking, 50, 106, 107
ankle rotations, 59, 108
appendicitis, 288, 289
appendix, 38, 85, 276
arches, 34–38
arguments, ending, 164–66
arms, 87, 111–12
    referral areas on, 43–45
arthritis, 222–24, 288, 289
asthma, 206–7, 209, 291
athletics, 241–54
    injuries and, 215, 243, 249–52
    "keeping eye on ball" in, 253
    muscle toning and, 248–49
    reflexology as part of regular training
        in, 243–47
    sleep and, 253
    visualization in, 253–54

back, 119, 290, 291
    disc problems and, 298, 299
    lower, 89, 90, 120, 230, 290
balls of feet, 32–34
bed rest, reflexology for children during,
    208–10
bedtime rituals, 211–13
bedwetting, 211–13, 290, 291
Bergman, William L., 10
big toes, 30–32, 271
bladder, 37, 41, 279
    problems of, 230, 233–34, 290, 291
    specific advice for, 84, 85, 86, 115, 118
blood pressure, 130
    high, 149–50, 236, 310, 311
    low, 149–50, 316, 317
bones, 274
    broken, 215, 251–52
    osteoporosis and, 179–80
Bowers, Edwin, 17
brain, 114, 271
breast-feeding, 179, 190
breasts, cysts or cancer in, 177–78, 292,
    293
breathing, 130, 139
breeze strokes, 63, 110, 122
broken bones, 215, 251–52
bronchial tube, 112
bronchitis, 292, 293
bruises, 215
buddy system, 264
Buonocore, Anthony, 9
bursitis, 292, 293
Byers, Dwight, 13, 48, 66

calcium, 26, 173, 179, 274
calluses, 292
cancer, 20, 100, 177–78
cardiovascular ailments, 236–38, 288,
    289
cataracts, 294, 295
cervical cancer, 177–78
chest area, 79–81, 111–12
childbearing, 181–91
    infertility and, 181–83, 312, 313
    labor in, 188–89
    postpartum recovery in, 189–91
    pregnancy in, 179, 183–88, 318, 319,
        322, 323

children, reflexology for, 20, 64, 193–
    217
    anatomy taught in, 198
    bedtime rituals and, 211–13
    broken bones or bruises and, 215
    common childhood illnesses and, 203
    communication opened by, 195–98
    confinement to bed and, 208–10
    fever and, 203–4
    foot problems and, 199
    hyperactivity or sluggishness and, 213–
        215
    infections and, 204–6
    introducing children to, 194–95
    newborns and, 190, 194–95, 199–200
    respiratory ailments and, 206–7
    skin irritations and, 201–2
    teenage turmoil and, 216–17
    teething and, 200
cholesterol, 294, 295
chronic area, 41, 90–91, 120
circulation, 18–19, 23, 26, 78, 94, 102,
    139, 171, 239, 249, 274, 275
colds, 20, 206–7, 294, 295
colitis, 294, 295
colon, 19, 37
    sigmoid, 38, 73, 84, 86, 115
    specific advice for, 84, 85, 86, 115,
        117
communication:
    of couples, 161–62
    of parents and children, 195–98
constipation, 230–33, 296, 297
couples, reflexology for, 152–67
    balance of power and, 166–67
    decision making and, 162–64
    ending arguments and, 164–66
    headaches, illness, or fatigue and,
        159–61
    lovemaking and, 152–55, 160
    sexual dysfunctions and, 156–59
    talking, sharing, or listening and,
        161–62
cramps, 94, 296, 297
    menstrual, 172–73, 318, 319
creams, 49
creativity, 20–21, 162–63
cross thumb slides, 62, 109
cystitis, 296, 297

decision making, 162–64
depression, 296, 297
diabetes, 224–26, 296, 297
diagnosing illnesses, 96
diaphragm, 81, 112, 277
diarrhea, 230–33, 298, 299
dieting, 261–63
digestive system, 130, 277, 278
disabled children, 208
disc problems, 298, 299
diverticulitis, 298, 299
dizziness, 298, 299
drug abuse, 216, 256, 257–59, 298, 299
drugs, before sessions, 95
dry skin (eczema), 300, 301
duodenum, 35, 118

earache, 300, 301
ears, 78, 113
eczema, 300, 301
edema, 234–36, 300, 301
elbows, 87, 243
emphysema, 300, 301
"empty nest syndrome," 163–64
endocrine system, 280
endorphins, 265
energy, 19–20, 94
    building up reserves of, 139–41
    too much or too little, in children, 213–15
energy zones, 21–23
epilepsy, 300, 301
eye disorders, 302, 303
    cataracts, 294, 295
    glaucoma, 304, 305
    vision loss and, 226–27
eyes, 78, 113
eye strain, 137–38

fainting, 302, 303
fallopian tubes, 41, 42, 281
    specific advice for, 92, 121
family, reflexology in, 198–99
fathers-to-be, 187
fatigue, 20, 26, 94, 135–36, 159–61, 220, 302, 303
feet:
    advice for specific parts of, 74–93
    checking for cuts, bruises, or calluses, 102, 105
    how to hold, 65–66
    locating specific points on, 29–30

as microcosm or mini-map of whole body, 24–25, 28–43
    perspiring of, 320, 321
    reasons for working with, 23–27
    sensitive tendon in, 29–30, 74, 82
    washing before sessions, 102–3
fever, 203–4, 302, 303
fight or flight response, 23, 129–31
fingertip rotations, 55, 107
fingertips, numbness in, 320, 321
finger walking, 70
fist slides, 61, 109
Fitzgerald, William, 17
five-toe rotations, 57
flatulence, 302, 303
flexing on a point, 72
fluid retention, 173, 234–36
foot boogie, 57, 108
fractures, 302
frigidity, 156

gallbladder, 35, 83, 118, 278
gallstones, 304, 305
glaucoma, 304, 305
gout, 304, 305
greeting feet, 49, 105, 106
groin, 41, 92, 93, 121
growths, abnormal, 304, 305
gum disorders, 326, 327

halitosis, 304, 305
hands, 87
    perspiring of, 320, 321
    referral areas on, 43–45
hanging on the ridge, 78, 79
happy hour, 134–35
hay fever, 306, 307
headaches, 159–61, 306, 307
head area, 75–76, 113–14
"healing crises," 94
health care professions, 283–84
hearing problems, 226–27, 306, 307
heart, 33, 111–12, 275
    problems of, 236–38, 288, 289
heart attacks, 147, 236, 308, 309
heartburn, 308, 309
heels, 34–38, 92–93
    spurs on, 326
hemorrhoids, 308, 309
hepatic flexure, 84, 117
hernias, 308, 309
herpes, 160

hiatal hernias, 308, 309
hiccoughs, 308, 309
high blood pressure, 149–50, 236, 310, 311
hips, 89–90, 120
    problems of, 310, 311
homeostasis, 19, 23, 280
hook and back-up, 73
hyperactivity, 195, 209, 213–15, 310, 311
hypertension (high blood pressure), 149–150, 236, 310, 311
hypoglycemia, 310, 311
hypotension (low blood pressure), 149–50, 316, 317
hypothalamus, 31, 73, 76, 114, 271
hysterectomy, 310, 311

ileocecal valve, 37, 73, 84, 85, 117
immune system, 20, 130, 131, 220, 276
    boosting, 144–46
impotence, 156, 312, 313
impurities, see toxins
incontinence, 312, 313
index finger slides, 52, 106
indigestion, 228–30, 312, 313
infection, 204–6, 312, 313
infertility, 181–83, 312, 313
influenza, 314, 315
Ingham, Eunice, 13, 17, 66
injuries, 243, 249–52
    broken bones, 215, 251–52
    to muscles, 249–50
inner foot, 38–39
insomnia, 211, 314, 315
intestines:
    small, 35, 37, 115, 117, 278
    see also colon
itchiness, 94

jaundice, 314, 315

karate chops, 63, 110
kidneys, 19, 37, 279
    problems of, 314, 315
    specific advice for, 84, 85, 115, 116, 118
kidney stones, 314, 315
knees, 89–90, 120
    problems of, 314, 315

labor, 188–89
laryngitis, 316, 317
"last chance syndrome," 163

learning disabilities, 196–97
leg bounce, 54, 107
legs, 89–90, 120
    problems of, 316, 317
leg stretch, 50, 105
Levy, Clifford B., 10
listening, couples' reflexology and, 161–162
liver, 34–35, 118, 278
    problems of, 266, 316, 317
lovemaking, 152–55, 160
low blood pressure, 149–50, 316, 317
lower back, 89, 90, 120, 230, 290
lower-back release, 50
lung press, 61, 109
lungs, 33, 111–12, 275, 277
lymph system, 19, 33–34, 276
    specific advice for, 80, 92, 93, 112, 121

mammary glands, 112, 281
medication, 95, 102
memory loss, 239–40
menopause, 175–77, 316, 317
menstruation, 172–75, 318, 319
metabolism, 265–66
midlife crises, 163
morning sickness, 183, 318, 319
motion sickness, 318, 319
muscles, 130, 242, 273, 274
    injuries to, 249–50
    toning, 248–49

nausea, 318, 319
neck area, 26, 77–79, 113
neck problems, 137–38, 318, 319
nervousness, 320, 321
nervous system, 23, 131, 271–72
neural pathways, 18
newborns, 190, 194–95, 199–200
numbness, in fingertips, 320, 321
nurturing, 160–61

older people, reflexology for, 219–40
    arthritis and, 222–24
    cardiovascular ailments and, 236–38
    diabetes and, 224–26
    edema and, 234–36
    elimination problems and, 230–34
    memory loss and, 239–40
    stomach problems and, 228–30
    vision or hearing problems and, 226–227
one-leg rocking, 54

one-leg stretch, 54, 107
open-heart surgery, 237
osteoporosis, 179–80
outer foot, 40
ovaries, 41, 42, 280, 281
    cysts or growths in, 177–78
    specific advice for, 92, 93, 121
over-the-ankle rotations, 59, 108

pains, sedentary, 137–38
palm rubdown, 56, 108
pancreas, 35, 116, 118, 224, 278, 280
Papa, Holly, 48
paralysis, 320, 321
parathyroids, 31, 78, 113, 280
perspiring, of hands or feet, 320, 321
Philbin, Regis, 100
phlebitis, 320, 321
pineal, 31, 271, 280
    specific advice for, 73, 76, 77, 114
pituitary, 31, 271, 280
    specific advice for, 73, 76, 77, 114
pivot on a point, 72
plastic surgery, 171
Plato, 129
pneumonia, 320, 321
polarity theory, 20
postpartum recovery, 189–91
power, balance of, 166–67
practitioners, rewards for, 21
pregnancy, 179, 181–88, 322, 323
    father's role in, 187
    infertility and, 181–83, 312, 313
    morning sickness during, 183, 318, 319
    physical ailments during, 183–86
    psychological ailments during, 186–187
    among teenagers, 217
premature ejaculation, 156
premenstrual syndrome (PMS), 173
preventive health care, 20, 129
productivity, 20–21
prostate, 41, 42, 230
    problems of, 322, 323
    specific advice for, 90, 92, 121
psoriasis, 322, 323
punching, 63, 110

rectum, 90, 120
referral areas, 43–45
reflexology:
    addictive behavior and, 255–66

advice for specific parts of foot in, 74–93
    athletics and, 241–54
    basic techniques in, 65–73
    benefits of, 16, 18–21
    for children, 20, 64, 190, 193–217
    clients' experiences during, 93–94
    for couples, 152–67
    general pointers for, 95–96
    health care professions and, 283–84
    history of, 17
    how to hold foot in, 65–66
    learning, 47–96
    methodology of, 21–23
    misinformation about, 27
    reasons for working with feet in, 23–27
    relaxation techniques in, 48–64, 95
    to strengthen body's systems, 269–81
    terminal illness and, 267–68
    for women, 169–92
    work or school and, 133–50
reflexology session order, 104–26
    alternate, 126
    chest, lung, heart, shoulder, and arm areas in, 111–12
    head area in, 113–14
    leg, knee, hip, and sciatic nerve areas in, 120
    neck, thyroid, and throat areas in, 113
    pelvic area to waist in, 115–17
    reflexing steps in, 111–21, 124–26
    relaxation steps in, 95, 105–10, 122, 123
    reproductive area in, 121
    spine and back area in, 119
    summary of, 123–26
    waist to diaphragm in, 118
reflexology sessions, 97–126
    for acne and skin disorders, 171–72
    for alcohol and drug abuse, 257–59
    for arthritis, 222–24
    for bedtime (especially for bedwetters), 212–13
    for bladder problems, 233–34
    for broken bones, 251–52
    for calming down, 147–48
    for communication with children, 198
    for constipation and diarrhea, 230–33
    for diabetes, 224–26
    for edema, 235–36
    for ending arguments, 165–66
    for energy reserves, 139–41
    environment for, 98–99

reflexology sessions (*cont.*)
  for eye, neck, and shoulder strain,
    137–38
  family, scheduling of, 199
  for fatigue, 135–36
  for feeling like equals, 166–67
  for fever, 203–4
  after game or workout, 245–47
  before game or workout, 243, 244–45,
    254
  for heart problems, 237–38
  for high or low blood pressure, 149–
    150
  for hyperactivity or sluggishness, 213–
    215
  for immune system, 144–46
  for indigestion, 228–30
  for infections, 204–6
  for infertility, 182–83
  for introducing children to reflexology,
    195
  during labor, 188–89
  for losing weight, 262–63
  for lovemaking, 154–55
  for memory improvement, 239–40
  for menopause, 175–77
  for menstrual regularity, 173–75
  for muscle injuries, 249–50
  for nervous system, 272
  for nurturing your partner, 161
  for older people, 221–22
  for osteoporosis, 179–80
  for ovarian or breast cysts and growths,
    177–78
  for postpartum recovery, 190–91
  for pregnancy difficulties, 184–86
  preparing for, 98–99, 102–4, 105
  questions asked during, 96
  for quitting smoking, 259–61
  for respiratory ailments, 206–7
  for sexual dysfunctions, 157–59
  for skin irritation, 201–2
  for someone confined to bed, 209–
    210
  for talking over serious issues, 162
  for teaching children about their
    bodies, 198
  for teething, 200
  for toning muscles, 248–49
  for travel stress, 142–43
  for vision or hearing losses, 226–27
  visualization techniques for, 100–101,
    104

relationships:
  nurtured by reflexology, 21
  see also couples, reflexology for
relaxation, 18, 23
  as antidote to stress, 131
  steps for, in session order, 105–10,
    122, 123
  techniques for, 48–64, 95
reproductive system, 41, 120, 121, 281
  see also childbearing; *specific organs*
respiratory ailments, 206–7
  asthma, 206–7, 290, 291
respiratory system, 277
"retirement syndrome," 220–21
reverse troughing, 53, 107
rotation on a point, 71

scar tissue, 249
school, reflexology and, 133–50
sciatica, 322, 323
sciatic nerve, 38, 41, 90–91, 120
scoliosis, 324, 325
sedentary aches and pains, 137–38
seminal vesicles, 41, 43, 92, 121, 281
seventh cervical vertebra, 32, 78, 79, 88,
  112
sex, 152–55, 160, 187
  teenagers and, 217
sexual dysfunctions, 156–59
  impotence, 156, 312, 313
sharing, couples' reflexology and, 161–
  162
shingles, 324, 325
shoes, for children, 199
shoulders, 111–12, 113
  pains in, 26, 324, 325
  strain of, 137–38
sibling rivalry, 198
sick days, reducing, 144–46
sigmoid colon, 38, 73, 84, 86, 115
sinuses, 113
sinusitis, 324, 325
skeletal system, 274
skin, 19, 170–72
skin disorders, 171–72, 324, 325
  acne, 171–72, 216, 287
  in children, 201–2
  eczema, 300, 301
  psoriasis, 322, 323
slapping, 63, 110
sleep, 163
  athletics and, 253
  insomnia and, 211, 314, 315

sluggishness:
  in children, 213–15
  see also fatigue
small intestines, 35, 37, 115, 117, 278
smoking, 259–61
solar plexus, 33, 271
  thumb press on, 51, 81, 106, 110, 122
sore throat, 326, 327
spinal cord, 271
spinal twist, 60, 109
spine, 24, 25, 38–39
  scoliosis of, 324, 325
  seventh cervical vertebra in, 32, 78, 79,
    88, 112
  specific advice for, 88–89, 112, 119
spleen, 35–36, 276
  specific advice for, 83, 84, 115, 116
sprains, 326, 327
spurs on heels, 326
stimulants, 102
stomach, 35, 116, 130, 278
  problems of, 228–30
stress, 18, 20, 23, 94, 127–31, 211, 275
  acne and, 216
  addictive behavior and, 256
  children and, 194
  detrimental effects of, 130
  facial signs of, 170–71
  fight or flight response to, 23, 129–31
  herpes and, 160
  infertility and, 181
  during pregnancy, 183, 186–87
  relaxation as antidote to, 131
  sexual dysfunctions and, 156
  time pressure and, 146–48
  of travel and vacations, 141–43
  at work or school, 134, 137
strokes, 147, 236, 326, 327
swelling, 26, 45
  edema and, 234–36, 300, 301

teenagers, 216–17, 264
teeth disorders, 326, 327
teething, 200
tennis elbow, 243
terminal illness, 267–68
testicles, 41, 42, 92, 93, 121, 280,
  281
thalamus, 271
thoracic area of spine, 112
throat, 113
  sore, 326, 327
thumb press, 51, 81, 106, 110, 122

thumb rotations, alternating, 53, 107, 110
thumb slides, 106
thumb walking, 67–69, 74
thymus, 112, 276, 280
thyroid, 31, 280
    specific advice for, 78, 112, 113
ticklishness, 48
time pressure, 146–48
tingling, 94
tinnitis, 326, 327
T-lymphocytes, 276
toe boogie, 58, 108
toe rotations, 108
toes, 25, 30–32, 271
    crooked or curled up, 75, 221
toe stretches, 58, 109
tonsillitis, 328, 329
tonsils, 276
toxins, 18, 19, 26, 94, 171, 173, 248, 266

travel stress, 141–43
troughing, 52, 106
    reverse, 53, 107
tumors, 328, 329
Type A vs. Type B personality, 147

ulcers, 328, 329
under-the-ankle rotations, 59, 108
ureters, 37, 84, 85, 115, 118, 279
urethra, 279
uric acid, 26
urinary system, 279
uterus, 41, 42, 90, 92, 121, 189

vacation stress, 141–43
vagina, 41, 281
varicose veins, 328, 329
vas deferens, 41, 43, 92, 281
vibrating, 53, 107
vision loss, 226–27

visualization techniques, 100–101, 104
    in athletics, 253–54
    for children, 195
vitality loss, 328, 329

walking, by babies, 199
weight loss, 261–63
whiplash, 80, 330
willpower, 266
women, reflexology for, 169–92
    cancer and, 177–78
    menopause and, 175–77
    menstrual problems and, 172–75
    osteoporosis and, 179–80
    skin care and, 170–72
    see also childbearing
work, reflexology and, 133–50
wringing, 62, 109

Zablozki, Vera, 11
zone theory, 17, 21–23